Dedication

To my amazing wife, **Bianca**—your love, patience, and unwavering belief in me have been my anchor through every storm. You are my strength, my peace, and my greatest blessing.

To my children and family—you are the reason I fight, the reason I rise, and the reason I never give up. Every step forward is for you.

To my close pals—thank you for always being there, for the laughs, the support, and the loyalty that money can't buy. You remind me that true friendship is priceless.

And to the best doctor in the world, my new best friend **Dr. HCK**—your skill, care, and compassion have given me more than health; you've given me hope. I owe you more than words can ever express.

To Andrew O'Callaghan, host of the mission critical podcast on Spotify, who gave me my voice and who continues to support me.

Thank you, my favourite Irishman.

This book is as much yours as it is mine. Without you all, this journey would not have been possible.

"STRENGTH IS NOT JUST WHAT WE CARRY ALONE—IT'S WHAT WE BUILD TOGETHER."

ALAN BATES

Foreword

This isn't a football hooligan book. It's not a glorified tale of terrace scraps or tribal warfare. It's a story about pain. About survival. About what happens when the fight moves from the streets into your own mind.

I grew up in a world where violence was normal, where loyalty was earned with fists, and fear was something you learned to bury deep. I was a rascal — wild, reckless, untouchable. I feared no man. I chased chaos like it was oxygen. But life doesn't care how tough you think you are. It finds a way to break you.

A rare and cruel disease came for me. No warning. No mercy. It stripped me down to the bone, left me hollowed out and drowning in despair. I planned my suicide with calm precision. I convinced myself it was the kindest thing I could do — for me, for my family, for anyone who'd ever cared. I made peace with the idea of disappearing.

But something stopped me. Something small. Something stubborn. A flicker of fight that refused to die.

This book is that flicker. It's not just my story — it's the story of men like me. Men who've worn the mask of strength for years. Men who've been told that talking is weakness, that emotion is shame, that silence is noble. Men who've battled depression in secret, who've stared down the barrel of suicide and lived to tell the tale.

These are tough men. Good men. Broken men. Brave men. And they all have one thing in common: they talk.

Real strength isn't silence. Real strength is standing in the storm and saying, "I NEED HELP." Real strength is choosing to live when dying feels easier. Real strength is speaking up — not just for yourself, but for the next man who's suffering in silence.

IF IT CAN HAPPEN TO ME

FROM THE TERRACES TO TRAUMA AND SURVIVAL

Alan Bates

Tough guys do talk. And it's time we shattered the myth that they don't.

My view on suicide is that you are ending your pain by handing it over to your loved ones, by baring my soul and the guest writers opening up, we are showing you that you are not alone and that the world is a better place with you in it.

CONTENTS

Dedication i

Foreword ii

Introduction: By Alberto Palmisciano 1

PART ONE 4

Chapter 1: N19 5DW — Born into the Smoke 5

Chapter 2: Two Up, Two Down 9

Chapter 3: Girdlestone Glory and Glue Sniffers 15

Chapter 4: Uncle Yid 18

Chapter 5: Take Your Laces Out, Son 21

Chapter 6: Red Bus Rover 27

Chapter 7: Guerra De La Malvinas 31

Chapter 8: Runaway 35

Chapter 9: If Anyone Runs 42

Chapter 10: I Met Stanley 47

Chapter 11: Unexpected Arrival 50

Chapter 12: Aunty Joan 55

Chapter 13: Villa Park 59

Chapter 14: Spud-U-Like 65

Chapter 15: The Pig & Whistle 72

Chapter 16: Do You Really Want to Hurt Me 79

Chapter 17: Micky Droy November '83 82

Chapter 18: Jasper Thompson 89

Chapter 19: Anderlecht's BCS 92

Chapter 20: More Than Just a Tear Up 96

PART TWO 103

Chapter 21: Bow Legged 104
Chapter 22: Dream Home 130
Chapter 23: Stalag 141
Chapter 24: Leave Me Alone 150
Chapter 25: Lokomat 152
Chapter 26: Universal Medical Centre Groningen 154
Chapter 27: Harry Helped Saved Me 168
PART THREE 175
Chapter 28: Introduction to the Stories of Strength 176
Chapter 29: James Ford (JT MOTIV) 212
Chapter 30: Beigal Bakery in Brick Lane 259
Chapter 31: Demons & Goals Colin W Chelsea Diver 276
Chapter 32: ADAM, MIND BODY&SOLE. 288
Chapter 33: DARRYL P. USA 294
Chapter 34: The Future for Alan Bates 297
Founder of TALK4STRENGTH 300
Support Contacts 304
Special Thanks 306

Introduction: By Alberto Palmisciano

On a rainy mid-March morning in Madrid, my mobile gave off a familiar 'bling' — another WhatsApp message. Nothing unusual. I get hundreds of them every week. I picked up the phone lazily, expecting the usual noise. But this one was different.

"Hi, my name is Alan Bates, and I got your number from a common friend in Frankfurt." A stranger. A Londoner. A Gooner. And he wanted to write a book.

He'd been told I had experience in the matter — fair enough, I've written a dozen books, mostly what people call "hoolie books," with the odd biography thrown in. I've helped others get their stories out too. I'm from a multicultural background, fluent in several languages, and I've written in Italian, Spanish, German, and English. But this wasn't about me. This was about Alan.

At first, I was ready to politely decline. But as Alan shared more, my curiosity grew. His main character was a lad from a rough London estate — the kind of place where fists speak louder than words, and football firms are family. He hinted at his past with Arsenal, then admitted he was Goner through and through. The firm might've flown under the radar compared to others, but they had their own code, their own battles, their own legacy.

Then came the gut punch. Alan told me about his current reality. He's living with a rare, degenerative disease — one that's slowly destroying his body while leaving his mind fully intact. There's no cure. No reprieve. Just a slow, merciless descent. He's 90% disabled. His brain, still sharp and defiant, refuses to accept the betrayal of his body. It's a daily war — not on the terraces, but within his own skin.

Alan sent me a podcast he recorded for The Mission Critical. I listened closely. For an hour, he spoke with raw honesty about his condition. His North London slang, his humour, his resilience — all barely masking the horror of what he endures. The list of symptoms was relentless. I felt the weight of it. I imagined myself in his shoes — and I crumbled. Alan lives it every day. And the worst is still ahead.

He told me his book would reflect this journey. That even the hardest hooligan — the kind who's stared down riot cops and rival firms — can be brought to his knees by illness. Vulnerability doesn't discriminate. And strength isn't just about fists and fury. It's about surviving when everything inside you screams to give up.

We spoke more. Alan knew his stuff. He'd lived the firm life from the inside. He knew the streets, the codes, the rivalries. He'd worked his way up in the building trade — from duct erector's mate to Construction Director. And now, he was facing the biggest fight of all: the one for his own life.

The more I learned, the more I respected him. I saw the fire in him. The grit. The refusal to be silenced. So, I jumped in. That's how I work — when a story grabs me, I dive in headfirst.

Alan reminded me of myself back in 2018, when I first tried writing. I'd spent years photographing riots at football matches across Europe — chasing chaos with a camera. It was risky. The police didn't like it. The hooligans liked it even less. But I did it anyway. I've got thousands of photos, many featured in the OLDSKOOL series. And when I finally sat down to write, I had no clue where to begin. A mate told me, "Just put pen to paper and let the memories flow." Seven years and a dozen books later, I can say that advice works. It's what I told Alan too.

Forget grammar and formatting — those can be fixed. What matters is the story. And Alan's story matters.

He's lived the firm life. He's fought the fights. He's earned the scars. And now, he's showing that even the toughest lads can break — and still find the strength to speak up. His book isn't just about football violence. It's about mental health, masculinity, and survival. It's about challenging the myth that silence equals strength.

Alan struggled to find international voices with street credibility to speak about clashes with the Gooners. That's why he reached out to me. Thanks to my OLDSKOOL work, I've connected with lads across Europe, and I was happy to help.

So here I am — a half-German, half-Italian, born in Belgium, living in Madrid — writing a foreword for a Londoner I've never met and may never meet. All because of a WhatsApp on a rainy Sunday.

Call it fate. Call it madness. I call it a little miracle, and I'm proud to be part of it.

PART ONE

Chapter 1: N19 5DW — Born into the Smoke

Our bath was made of tin and sat on the roof of the outside khazi. Us Londoners call it a khazi — most would know it as a toilet. But this wasn't some quaint outdoor loo with a garden view. It was a freezing, cobweb-ridden box that stank of bleach and piss, perched like an afterthought behind the house. The bath was dragged out when needed, filled with kettles and pans, and emptied with buckets. Luxury didn't live here.

I wasn't born into comfort. I was born into concrete. Into chaos. Into a part of London that the city forgot — a slum tucked between crumbling old houses and piss-stained alleyways, where the only thing that came easy was trouble.

I was born in the Archway — a rough old gaff in the north of the London Borough of Islington. In the 1960s, it was a patchwork of slums, most marked for demolition but still stuffed with families. Five of us crammed into two upstairs rooms in a house with a shared kitchen. The walls were thin, the floors creaked like they were begging for mercy, and the cold seeped into your bones like a second skin.

Kids played football with half-flat balls in the street that doubled as battlegrounds. The older lads smoked, spat, and sized each other up, someone was always looking for a fight, you learned fast — or you got flattened.

Archway was rough, the kind of place where you learned to fight before you learned to read.

The name itself came from the bridge that loomed over the area, known locally as Suicide Bridge. Not just a nickname — a warning. That bridge had seen more tragedy than most care to admit. It cast a long shadow, both literally and metaphorically, over the lives below.

There's the legend of Dick Whittington, the merchant who came to London from Gloucestershire to learn the trade of a Mercer. He became Lord Mayor of London four times, and the story goes that he paused on Highgate Hill, looked out over the city, and heard the Bow bells ringing. That sound, they say, makes you a true Cockney. As I didn't know that story until very much later in life, whenever someone called me a Cockney, I'd correct them — I'M NOT A COCKNEY, but ultimately, I was born and bred in the shadow of those bells, so all of us Archway bods are indeed COCKNEYS.

Our rooms were box rooms in the upstairs of an old terraced house.

The heating was a gas fire that my mum always lit her fags from. You could hear every argument through the paper-thin walls — couples screaming, babies crying, Privacy didn't exist. Peace didn't either.

It couldn't have been easy for my mum and dad, but like everyone else in the area, we got by. You didn't complain — you cracked on. You didn't dream — you survived. The area was a jungle of noise, fights, and families stitched together by hardship. The smell of coal smoke, chip shops, and damp brick was constant. You could taste the poverty in the air.

My dad, Donald Alfred Bates, was born in Middlesex — now North London. His bloodline ran through St Pancras, Edmonton, and Bethnal Green. East End stock. He did his national service in 1951, two years in the British Army. That was the law back then — every young man trained to defend Britain if called upon. It gave them discipline, but it also gave them stories.

He told me about arriving in Aldershot for training. A bunch of 18-year-olds, fresh off the estates, lined up like mannequins on the tarmac. Names were called. When your name came, you stepped forward. My dad's name was called. "You ugly bunch are going to Germany," barked the sergeant. Relief. He knew what the other option was. Then came the rest: "You fine gentlemen will be going to Korea." Silence. Those lads were headed to a war halfway across the world. A brutal, three-year conflict that claimed over 1,100 British lives.

Dad got lucky. He went to Germany, became a lorry driver, and spent most of his time ferrying army prisoners between barracks and the military jail in Bielefeld. But luck has limits. While he was stationed there, his mum died — just 40 years old.

After dad's national service he arrived home to find a stranger opening the door to his parents' house. His dad had remarried. The new wife didn't want him there. No welcome. No warmth. Just rejection. His own father — a man I refuse to call grandad — had moved on without a second thought.

My mum was a Londoner too, but her roots were different. Her parents came from the Northeast — land of the coal mines. My grandad, David Pickles, was an illiterate miner. No shame in that. These men didn't need books — they needed backbone. Born in Oakenshaw, Durham, he worked at Chop well Colliery and started out as a pony driver for the Consett Iron Co. He was tough, quiet, and friendly.

Then he met Minnie Tyers. What a name. Minnie Tyers — soon to be Minnie Pickles. She was educated, came from a slightly higher-class family, but still tied to the colliery. Her dad, Tommy Tyers, wasn't thrilled about the match. A miner and his daughter? Not on his watch. But love doesn't ask for permission. David and Minnie ran away together, eloped, and boarded a train heading south.

The trains from Durham went north or south. North offered more pits. The South offered London — the beating heart of the empire. They chose London. Arrived at King's Cross, found a room in Islington, and started a family. Nine kids. Nine loud, proud, scrappy kids. That Geordie blood mixed with London grit created some characters. My aunts and uncles were legends — and lunatics. Family gatherings were loud, messy, and often ended in punch-ups. That was normal. That was love.

School was a joke. Teachers were knackered, classrooms overcrowded, and half the kids were already halfway to becoming criminals. You didn't go there to learn — you went to survive. I got into punch-ups before I could spell my own name. Respect was earned with fists, with fear, with how many lads you could make flinch when you walked past.

The streets were ruled by unspoken laws. You didn't grass. You didn't cry. You didn't back down. If someone looked at you wrong, you stared back harder. If someone shoved you, you swung. Weakness meant that you would soon become a victim.

We didn't have much, but what we had, we protected. Our mates, our turf, our name. You didn't need money to have honour. You just needed backbone.

That's where I came from. Not the glossy London you see on postcards. Not the posh bits with cafés and cobblestones. I came from the underbelly. The forgotten corners. The places where boys became men too fast, and some didn't make it at all.

And that's where the fight started. Not in the terraces. Not in the firms. But in the grime, the grit, the grind of growing up in a world that didn't give a toss if you lived or died.

Chapter 2: Two Up, Two Down

As a kid, I was just the same as all the others, black, Irish, Greek, Turkish, we all stuck together — and I loved every second of it.

I'd sit on the front step, knees scuffed, nose running, watching the older lads square up in the street. No rules, no refs, just raw aggression. You could smell the tension before the first punch landed — a mix of sweat, chip grease, and adrenaline. They didn't fight for money or pride. They fought for respect. For turf. For the right to walk down the road without being looked at sideways.

To me, they were Legends. I'd watch wide-eyed as fists flew and swearwords that fascinated me. Blood was just part of the show. A badge of honour. If you walked away with a split lip and your head held high, you'd earned your place. I wanted that. I never wanted to be feared, but I wanted to be respected, but for now, I was just a kid — soaking it all in, storing it for later.

The streets were cracked and crooked, the buildings still scarred from the war. You could see it in the bricks — blackened patches where fire had burned the walls, jagged edges where bombs had torn through homes. The older folk didn't talk about it much, but you could feel it. The silence was heavy. Like the city itself was still holding its breath.

My mum used to tell me stories about the German bombing raids. How the sirens would scream through the night, how families would scramble into shelters clutching blankets and babies. She said that the scariest thing that she ever heard and it haunted her all her life was when Hitler's doodle bugs stopped squealing, because you knew that it would fall out of the sky and it would be close by or on top of you.

She would say the sky lit up like hell had opened its gates. She'd seen buildings collapse like sandcastles, neighbours just disappear, and firemen cry as they pulled bodies from rubble. She was just a girl then — but she remembered everything.

Don and Jean, Paul, Donna and I made up the Bates family.

When I was two years old, my mum and dad got the letter from the council — we were being given a three-bedroom flat in a big old red brick estate on Brecknock Road. Now that was some place. Built in 1938, it had survived the Blitz, the bombs, and the chaos of war. On Black Saturday, September 7th, nearly 1,000 German bombers and fighter escorts tore through London. Islington got pummelled. 430 killed. 1,600 injured. But somehow, the red brick stood firm. Mr. Hitler threw everything he had at it, and it didn't flinch.

Imagine how my mum felt — stepping into that flat. A proper bathroom with a bath. A kitchen she didn't have to share. And best of all, a toilet indoors. No more freezing your arse off at the bottom of the garden. No more tin baths on the roof. You could have a pony in the warm. That must've felt like heaven. After years of grime and graft, she had her own space. Her own throne. She walked through that flat like a queen. Chin up. Shoulders back. Curtains hung like silk. Floors scrubbed like marble. That bathroom wasn't just porcelain — it was pride.

Life on the estate was electric. A melting pot of kids — Black, white, mixed race, Irish, Greek, Turkish — all running wild together. We were the red brick kids. From the Brecknock. sixteen blocks, one middle drive, and a thousand stories.

We lived on the third floor in 215 Morris House. According to my mum, if you wanted to find our flat, you just followed the trail of blood up the stairs — that was Alan's house. If it wasn't swings cracking my skull while we tried to wrap them round the top bar, it was stone fights, bike crashes, or falling off walls. The best one? A tug-of-war with an old pushbike innertube. Those things could stretch like hell. I had this genius idea — let go at full stretch and Peter would get a sore hand. Turns out he had the same idea. We both let go. BOOM. I got caught as always.

The valve — the one you pump air through — jammed itself between my knuckles. Proper stuck. I ran home, blood spurting, and mum yanked it out. Wrapped it up. Sent me back out laughing about the new hole in my hand. Still got the scar fifty years later.

The middle drive was our Berlin Wall. You didn't cross it unless you had backup. The older kids ruled it. They'd stand you against the wall and take turns booting footballs at you. Set their dogs on you — not to bite, just to scare. All the usual post-war council estate hospitality.

My brother Paul was eight years older. One day, him and his mates were chucking rocks at clay drainpipes during some building work. They stood the pipe on a pile of sand. When it got knocked over, guess who had to run up and stand it back up? Yep. Little Al. I'm halfway up the mound when a rock smashes the pipe. I grab the new piece, climb to the top, and BOSCH — I'm knocked off with blood pumping everywhere.

Paul's shouting at the kid who threw it. I'm clutching my face, blood dripping off my elbows. Panic sets in. They don't know if it's hit my eye. They're not worried about me — they're worried about what mum will do. Excuses fly. Stories form. Eventually, Paul takes me upstairs and tells mum I fell off the swings. Jean's not having it. She patches me up, gives me a bollocking, then cuddles me and feeds me chocolates for days. That was the way — you got told off, patched up, and loved hard. And Paul? Got away with it. Typical. He'll swear blind he doesn't remember it. But I do, mate. I remember it all.

There was a rumour going round — lads from an estate near Holloway, right by the women's prison, were coming to fight the Brecknock boys. Bad move. Our estate had lunatics. Even the birds could fight. It was like the council had picked the maddest families and thrown them all into the red brick.

We were just kids — seven or eight — and found a patch of grass on a hill not covered in dog shit. Prime viewing spot. The middle drive was the battlefield. Both sides of the estate joined forces. The other lads came down the hill. Their top boy squared up to ours. His sister stood beside him — Susan. They talked. We watched. Then BOOM — our lad headbutted theirs. Missed his face, caught his collarbone. It popped out. Screaming. Chaos. Susan went Garrity — swinging at anyone she didn't recognise. She was wild. Years later, when I read about Boudica and Viking shield maidens, I thought of her. She'd have led armies.

Growing up in the inner cities of the UK in the 60s and 70s was as tough as it gets. School fights. Estate fights. Area fights. Mods vs Skinheads. Skins vs Punks. Football vs everyone.

One day, I was playing football in the washing drying area — murder ball, keepy-uppys, loving life. Then a group of Black kids surrounded me. Fear kicked in. One lad poked me in the chest. I was crying. His big brother shouted, "Hit him! He hit you — hit him back!" Turns out a blond kid had smacked him earlier. They came looking. Found the wrong blond kid. Me.

I froze. Proper terrified. My sister Donna was on the balcony. She saw me — her little brother, paralysed with fear. Now, Donna's only 4ft 11 as an adult.

She is tiny, but God made her in a tiny package to protect others, Donna fears no one. I love her with every beat of my heart, but fuck me, I was scared of her. In through the crowd of kids burst my big sister. The kid was still pushing and eager to fight, but he was not getting his way because I just stood crying. My sister screamed at me, if you don't hit him back, I will bash you. I have never feared many people, but my sister has always been someone that puts the wind up me, so as soon as the kid pushed me that last time, boom I went ballistic.

While punch up and scars were part of everyday life, football hadn't yet entered my bloodstream. At five years old, I didn't understand the tribalism, the hatred, the obsession. I knew what a ball was. I knew how to kick it. But I didn't know what it meant.

That changed on Monday evening, the 3rd of May, 1971.

The estate erupted. The noise was unreal — like a bomb had gone off, but instead of panic, there was joy. Pure, unfiltered joy. People were hugging strangers, kissing in the streets, dancing on balconies. Flags waved from windows. Scarves hung from lampposts. Bed sheets with player names were draped over railings. The red brick estate — usually full of shouting, fighting, and chaos — was now a cathedral of celebration.

Arsenal had just won the league. And they'd done it at White Hart Lane.

I didn't understand the gravity of it then. I didn't know that winning the title on your rival's turf was the ultimate insult, the sweetest victory. But I felt it. I felt the energy. The pride. The unity. For once, the estate wasn't divided by scraps or postcode beef — it was united in red and white.

The next morning, it was like Christmas. Flags everywhere. Scarves tied to railings. Kids running around chanting. Adults still buzzing from the night before. The estate was only a half-hour walk from Highbury, so you can imagine — the whole area was alive. It wasn't just a win. It was a moment. A memory. A marker in time.

Then came the big one.

Saturday, 8th of May 1971. Arsenal vs Liverpool. FA Cup Final. If Arsenal won, it would be their first ever double — league champions and FA Cup winners in the same season. History in the making.

The buzz on the estate was electric. Everyone was talking about it. Radios were tuned in. TVs were ready. And for us, it was personal. Charlie George — the hero of the Arsenal faithful — grew up on the estate next door. He went to Holloway School, just 200 yards from the red brick. He was one of us. A local lad. A Brecknock boy. And now, he was about to write his name in football folklore.

The match kicked off. Ninety minutes passed — 0-0.
Tension everywhere. Then Steve Heighway scored for
Liverpool. The air shifted. You could hear "You'll Never Walk
Alone" echoing from every pub and living room. But the red
brick didn't flinch. We held our breath. And then — BOOM —
Eddie Kelly scrambled in the equaliser. The estate exploded.
Chants rang out:

"CHAMPIONS! CHAMPIONS!" "GOOD OLD
ARSENAL!" "WE'RE PROUD TO SAY THAT NAME!"
"ARSENAL! ARSENAL! ARSENAL!"

And then it happened. Charlie George. The boy from Brecknock Road. King Charlie hit the winner.

The celebration was biblical. People cried. People screamed. People ran into the streets like it was the end of the war. I didn't fully grasp what had happened — not yet — but I knew it was special. I knew it mattered. I knew that football wasn't just a game. It was identity. It was pride. It was war without bullets.

We lived on the Brecknock until I was nine. I loved it. Every scar, every fight, every laugh. It was home. And then, just like seven years earlier, the letter arrived from the council.

Another move. Another chapter. But the red brick? That was where it all began.

Chapter 3: Girdlestone Glory and Glue Sniffers

I never knew, but where they'd knocked all the slums down in Archway, they built a brand-new estate — one of the biggest ever thrown up in the borough of Islington. Concrete blocks, fresh brick, new layouts. It was like someone had taken a wrecking ball to the past and tried to build a future.

My mum had been a constant pain in the arse to the rent office down Elthorne Road. She was relentless — letters, visits, complaints. She didn't ask for better housing, she demanded it. And it worked. One day, the letter dropped through the letterbox. We'd been allocated a brand spanking new three-bedroom maisonette.

We'd gone from two rooms with an outside khazi and a shared kitchen, to a pre-war flat with a bathroom and our own kitchen. And now — wait for it — we had two toilets. Two khazis. Can you believe it? In the space of seven years, we'd gone from boiling kettles for a tin bath to flushing from two separate karzees. We felt like royalty, when my brother and sister left home, I had the upstairs bedroom and it had its own toilet.

Its sounds like I'm obsessed with toilets, doesn't it.

161 Girdlestone Walk. Bredgar Road. London N19 5DW. Two balconies. Two toilets. A kitchen big enough for a table where the whole family could sit together. The Bates`s had struck gold.

We were the first to move into the block. Over the next few months, the estate started to fill up — new faces, new families, new noise. The racial mix was still there, but most of the white kids were Irish. We didn't clock it at the time, other than noticing their schools always started with "Saint this" or "Saint that."

Underneath the flats, they'd built garages — one for each flat, available for a small weekly fee. It was modern. It was clever but It was doomed. The glue sniffers soon turned the garages into dens of madness. They'd smash the lights; pry open the doors by tugging from the bottom until they bent like tin foil and sit in the dark with crisp bags full of Evo-Stik. One sniff and they were off — high as kites, eyes glazed, mouths slack. It got so bad; the council bricked up entire garage blocks within the first year. So much for modern design.

The move meant a new school for me. Hargrave Park Primary, right at the top of the road. My first day was a baptism of fire. Three kids grabbed me — one on each arm, the third booting me in the shins. "Does that hurt?" he asked. Course it fucking hurt. But I said "No." So he kept kicking. Over and over. Until a teacher finally saw and broke it up.

I hated those three. Especially the kicker. His face is still burned into my memory. If I saw him today, I'd still hate him. But the other two? Absolute characters. Funny, cheeky, proper little troublemakers. I ended up liking them. There's something about naughty kids — they always seem older than they are. More streetwise. Into things way beyond their years. The only thing I couldn't stand? They were Spurs fans.

The school itself was one of those old brick buildings built in the early 1900s. And in the early 1970s, the headmaster was proper old school. Mr Lashbrook. A man who believed punishment should fit the crime. If you got caught spitting, you sat outside his office with a bucket and spat into it until home time. The bucket never filled and home time never came fast enough.

If you got into a fight, you sorted it out with gloves on. No messing. No sulking. You got in the ring and handled it. On one of the lower floors, between the juniors and the infants, Mr L had a full boxing ring set up. Every Tuesday morning, while the rest of the school were in assembly singing hymns and pretending to be angels, us lads were down there smashing the granny out of each other.

And here I am, writing this in 2025, knowing there are nine-year-olds out there identifying as cats — while we were strapping on gloves the size of our heads and knocking lumps out of each other. Different times.

Each year, there was an end-of-term boxing night. Parents came. Kids got paired off by size. And we fought. Proper fights. No headgear. No mercy. I'll never forget mine. My dad and brother came to watch. I was up against Dele L — an African kid, a monster of a boy.

Anyway, I got paired against D — and you could almost see him licking his lips in the other corner, like a lion eyeing up a lamb chop. He was built like an African buffalo, all muscle and menace, and I was the sacrificial offering.

The bell went. And then it started.

D's long, muscly arms were everywhere — pop, pow, bong — it was like watching an episode of BATMAN AND ROBIN. You remember those scraps with the Joker or the Penguin, where the screen flashed up with words like BIFF, BASH, BANG? Well, those words were exploding in my head every time he landed a shot.

I did my best. I kept my gloves up. I moved. I ducked. I took the hits. Other than a nosebleed, I held my ground. I didn't crumble. I didn't cry. I didn't quit.

I was never going to win — everyone knew that. But I showed up. I stood tall. And in that ring, under those lights, in front of my dad and my brother, I did myself proud.

Sometimes, it's not about winning. It's about proving you belong. And that day, I did.

Chapter 4: Uncle Yid

My Uncle Tommy used to take me over to Tottenham to watch the football. Uncle Tom was a proper character — funny, sharp, with a dry sense of humour that could cut through any silence. I loved him dearly. He had that old-school charm, the kind that made you feel safe even when you were somewhere you didn't belong.

Tommy's best mate Joe was an Arsenal fan. From what I understand, back in the 1950s and 60s, it wasn't uncommon for pals to support different clubs and still go to football together every Saturday. Arsenal one week, the vermin the next — whoops, I meant Spurs. Strange to think about now, because by the time I was growing up, mixing with them was rare. You picked your side and stuck to it.

When Uncle Tommy was cremated, the piano rolled into GLORY GLORY TOTTENHAM HOTSPUR. The whole crematorium filled with that anthem. People looked around at me — some laughing through tears, others just shaking their heads. It was a moment. A tribute. A send-off. The family told me that whenever my name came up, Tommy would say, "You do know he was Tottenham before he was Arsenal." I never held it against him. He was family. And he was a good man.

Anyway, back to the two rowdy schoolmates. When I was a pup, you could go to Arsenal or Spurs and just pay on the door. No memberships, no digital tickets, no nonsense. These two Herberts asked if I fancied going to a Spurs v Arsenal game. We jumped on the 41 buses at Archway and off we went — straight to the swamp. Never a more apt name, in my opinion.

I was in the Spurs lot. They were winning. The atmosphere was electric — addictive, even. The joy and venom oozing from the crowd was both fascinating and exhilarating. They were singing songs about kicking people's heads in, about sending you home in a blood-stained ambulance. It was mental. It was exciting beyond belief. It was fun — until it wasn't.

Because I wasn't a Spurs fan. In fact, even at that age — 11 or 12 at most — I already hated them.

I got separated from my mates during the celebrations. Alone. Surrounded by the enemy. I didn't know yet that they'd become my lifelong rivals, but I knew I didn't belong there. I couldn't stand it. The songs, the faces, the smugness. It made my skin crawl.

So, all I had to do was get my head down and walk up the High Road to the bus garage and get on the 41 bus back to the Archway, that bus would drop me off within a 5-minute walk to my mum & dads.

As I left the ground, an older bloke started chatting to me. "You got the fucking hump as well, mate?" he asked. "Yeah," I replied. "I was in with their lot, and got separated. Couldn't stand it."

We walked together, chatting. He seemed like a good bloke, he was — probably late teens or early twenties. But then he went quiet. Across the road, near a little monument where the road splits toward Walthamstow, sat five or six Spurs fans. Skinheads. Rude boys. You could tell they hadn't been at the match. The radio would've told them Spurs were winning. They were waiting — like hyenas — ready to pick off stragglers. Bully tossers.

We put our heads down. Tried to walk past. My new mate leaned in and said, "When they get near, just run. Run as fast as you can."

They stepped onto the pavement. "Hello mate, you been to the football?" one of them asked.

And all I heard was: **RUN. RUN. RUN.**

So, I did. Legs pumping, heart thumping. They weren't interested in me — I was just a kid. But the punches started flying immediately. My new mate took a proper kicking. The poor fucker. A bloke on his own, getting caned by a group of lads. How brave is that?

That moment stuck with me. The cruelty. The pack mentality. The way they hunted. It was football, yes — but it was something darker too.

Growing up on an estate where you could jump on the 41 to the swamp or any bus down Holloway Road to Highbury meant you were always in the mix. There were Spurs fans on the estate. Around the area. You knew who they were. You clocked them. You didn't always fight — but you never forgot.

And me? I'd seen enough. I knew where I stood. I was Arsenal. Forever.

Chapter 5: Take Your Laces Out, Son

Andy Briton was a kid on our estate. A proper goalkeeper — reminded me of Peter Shilton. Every time we played football, he was diving all over the place like his life depended on it. His dad, Charlie, was a top bloke. Staunch Chelsea fan. They used to take me to Stamford Bridge, and every other week we'd stand in the Shed — to the right as you looked at the pitch.

By then, I'd properly caught the football bug. I was willing to go anywhere to watch a match. And when it kicked off — inside or outside the stadium — I wasn't scared. I was buzzing. Sounds mad even writing it now, but it's true. I wasn't involved, but the chaos excited me. It was like theatre — violent, tribal, unpredictable theatre.

Chelsea's home end was called the Shed. In fairness, it wasn't much more than a shed. But the boys sang their hearts out. In those days, Chelsea were pony — the ground rarely full. But if there were a decent number of away fans, the Shed boys would belt out:

"North Stand, North Stand, do your job!"

The North Stand was opposite the Shed. A weird setup — high at the back, sloping down like a hill. Away fans were dumped at the bottom. The North Stand boys would gather at the top and charge down like warriors. Fencing or not, there was always a chance they'd get at each other.

After the final whistle, you'd shuffle out with the crowd. And sometimes, it was mayhem. Police horses charging up and down. Coppers shouting. Skinheads in shiny DMs, stay-pressed trousers with neat turn-ups, Harrington jackets or sheepskin coats. They looked mean. Menacing. Like they'd been bred for violence.

They'd wait for the away fans to be let out, then move like sharks smelling blood. Down toward Fulham Broadway station, just as the away fans spilled out. The old bill had no chance. In those days, the kozzas would just bash you. Horses cracking skulls. Foot coppers swinging batons like Bruce Lee with nun chucks. "Get back! Get back!"

What fascinated me was how the hooligans knew who they wanted. If you didn't want it, you moved away. But the like-minded away fans stepped forward — and boom, it was on. Men fighting back and forth. Hotdog stands getting flattened. The smell of horse shit in the air. The roar of the crowd. It was chaos. It was tribal. It was beautiful.

A mate on the estate — lived opposite me — was a Leeds fan. Yeah, I know. A Leeds fan in London. Lived 4.8 miles from Tottenham, 1.9 from Arsenal. But he chose Leeds. Go figure.

"Al, do you fancy going to Ipswich with Leeds?" Didn't need asking twice. I had my DMs on and couldn't wait.

Off we popped to Liverpool Street station for a proper adventure. When we got there, it was a sight — gangs of lads in white and yellow scarves, DM boots, and a look that was hard to describe. Not like the Chelsea boys. These lot had more hair. My mate Keiran G clearly knew people. We walked over to a rowdy, cocky, intimidating bunch of Leeds fans — but they sounded like us. No strange accents. Turns out Leeds had a mob called the Cockney Whites.

Keiran's Account: IPSWICH AWAY.

It was during the 76/77 season. I used to travel — when pocket money allowed — with the London Leeds Supporters Club. Home games were a slog. Over three hours each way. 9:10am from King's Cross to Leeds, back around 10pm. So, I preferred away games — especially the five London clubs in the First Division.

One day in '76, my mate and neighbour Alan Bates asked if he could come to a game out of town. He'd heard my Sunday stories — not just about football, but the off-pitch antics. Fights inside and outside the ground. Station tear ups, the lot.

On November 20th, 1976, Alan and I told our parents we were heading to the West End for Christmas shopping. I told my mum I didn't fancy the Ipswich game — chance of a frozen pitch — just in case it came up later.

We met my schoolmate David Crockett and headed to Liverpool Street. Got our tickets (£1.50) from the club secretary and boarded the train with 25–30 Cockney Whites. The journey was full of banter, trivia, and a few morning bevvies — Coca-Cola for us, we were still kids.

We arrived in Ipswich around lunchtime and broke into the customary away fan chant:

"London Leeds, we are here — oh oh!"

Alan, being a lifelong Arsenal fan, understandably didn't join in.

It was freezing. I was jealous of Alan's 10-hole steel toe cap Docs. I had Adidas Roms — my feet were blocks of ice. But envy turned to awe when we got to the turnstiles. A copper — possibly the biggest in Suffolk — stood on Alan's toes.

"Are they steels?" he asked. "Yes," Alan replied. "Take your laces out, son."

He handed Alan a luggage tag. Alan wrote his address on it. The laces were to be collected after the match. Steel toe caps were seen as weapons — removing the laces was meant to stop you using them.

Inside, the atmosphere was electric. Full house. Away fans packed into one half of the stand behind the goal, separated from the Ipswich lot by wire mesh and a line of coppers. We were at the top of the terrace — six feet from the enemy. Singing, shouting, taunting. It was glorious.

Ipswich equalised with 15 minutes to go — chasing Liverpool and Man City for the title. Ironically, the goal was scored by Brian Talbot, who'd later become an Arsenal favourite.

After the goal, Dave Crockett climbed onto the roof stanchions above the police line, taunting the Ipswich fans with:

"You're going to win fuck all!"

They replied with:

"We're going to win the league!"

It was loud. It was wild. It was perfect.

Kieren G

Back to my memory of the trip, we boarded the train and off we went — seats found, buzz building, the carriage alive with accents and banter. But the person getting all the attention wasn't some geezer in a Stone Island jacket. It was a bird. Dressed head-to-toe in double denim, smoking like a chimney, drinking like a docker, and barking orders like she ran the firm.

She sounded rough — proper rough. Like a bear's arse with a sore throat. But she had a presence. Command. And respect. Turns out she was a well-known face in the Leeds firm. Not just tolerated — revered. She was the matriarch of mayhem, and no one dared cross her.

The train — or the rattler, as we called it — rolled toward Ipswich. Everyone expected the Ipswich firm to be waiting on the platform, ready for a scrap. Doors were opening before the train even stopped. Lads desperate to be first out, to steam into the home mob. The adrenaline was infectious.

The rattler screeched to a halt. Roars went up: **"UNITED! UNITED!"**

But there was no Ipswich firm. Just a wall of Suffolk Constabulary — the finest stick-wielding farmers in uniform.

Leeds had a fierce reputation. The police weren't taking chances. They wrapped us up like cattle and marched us to the ground. No freedom. No chaos. Just a slow, controlled shuffle through the streets.

At the turnstiles, the old bill was checking boots. If you had DMs, you were fucked.

"Take your laces out, son." "What? What for?" **"Just take your laces out."**

I was just a kid. What was I going to do — launch a flying kick into the Ipswich end? **"TAKE YOUR FUCKING LACES OUT!"**

I obliged. The next step was clearly a clip round the ear from a copper who sounded like he'd just come off a tractor. My feet were freezing. But not as bad as the poor sods in steel toe caps — they had their boots confiscated and were left standing in their socks. It was like a scene from a prison yard.

The match itself was eye-opening but uneventful. The real drama came after — back at King's Cross underground station. Saturday evening. Dangerous territory. Any mob from any club could be lurking. You had to keep your head on a swivel.

We were just kids. Trying to look the part. Trying to get into hooliganism. But truth be told, we were just making up the numbers. Watching. Learning. Soaking it all in.

Then we saw them — a group of football lads walking toward us. "Hello boys," one of them said. "Where are you from?"

Phew. Cockney accent. "The Archway."

"So, you're Arsenal?" "No, we aren't into football." "What are you doing here then? Dressed like little thugs?"

We were fucked.

“Do you know who we are?” “No.”

“We’re Cockney Reds.”

Thank fuck Keiran didn’t say he was Leeds. Man United’s Cockney Reds hated Leeds with a passion.

Then the main bully piped up: **“Liverpool Cockney Reds — not those Manc cunts.”**

We still didn’t know what they were going to do. The tension was thick. Then, out of nowhere, a sound — loud, rhythmic, growing closer. A gang of men chanting, marching toward our platform. We couldn’t make out the words, but we knew there were loads of them.

The Cockney Reds absolutely shit themselves. And like a puff of magic dust — they vanished.

Then the group arrived. Singing like a Welsh men’s choir. Drunken. Loud. Joyful.

Phew. They were Welsh rugby fans. Didn’t even know we existed.

Fuck knows what they were doing on our platform. But they were well lost. And they saved our bacon.

Chapter 6: Red Bus Rover

It was a beautiful Saturday. The sun is shining. Streets buzzing. A few of us decided to get a red bus rover ticket — 50p for adults, 25p for kids. That little slip of paper gave you access to every red London bus for 24 hours. Value for money? Unbeatable.

We had no plan. Just the freedom to roam. For some reason, we ended up in South London — Greenwich Park, the observatory, the Cutty Sark. Tourist stuff. But one of the older lads with us was a West Ham fan, and they were playing at Charlton. So, he said, "Let's go to the game."

We jumped on the next bus heading toward Woolwich. Sirens everywhere. Blue lights flashing. The tension was rising before we even saw the floodlights.

And then they came into view — towering above the rooftops like beacons. For me, floodlights always meant excitement. Football. Atmosphere. Chaos.

It was September 21st, 1976. A day many would never forget. A day that ended in tragedy.

Before the game, the atmosphere was strange. The police looked rattled — overwhelmed by the sheer number of young men milling about, not just loitering, but actively hunting for trouble. It wasn't the usual away-day vibe. This was different. Very different.

Normally, away fans stuck together. But here, it was fractured. People were starting on each other, and you couldn't tell who was who.

We got into the ground — the most packed stadium I'd ever seen. It was intense. Fighting broke out everywhere. Not where we were — we were in the West Ham away section — but all around us, it was kicking off.

The game started. Then, like clockwork, the roar went up from the Charlton stand — the Undercover End.

"UNITED! UNITED!"

A gap opened up. West Ham were on the right-hand side of the stand. Charlton fans who wanted it made their way toward the open space. And then it started — fists flying, bodies crashing, chaos erupting.

They said 50,000 were squeezed into the ground. Official attendance? 35,000. But in those days, you could jump turnstiles or slip the bloke a quid and he'd let you in. No scanners. No stewards. Just nods and winks.

West Ham won the game. Jubilation. But outside, it was carnage.

Pushing. Shoving. Police horses charging. Coppers swinging batons at anyone in reach — innocent or not.

We later found out a young man had been kicked into a coma.

We didn't know the area. We just followed the West Ham fans, assuming they were heading to the station. I was 11. Not scared of the fighting — at that age, you think you've got a force field around you. But I was tired. I'd been out since morning. It was getting dark. And I was deep in South London as they say — bandit country.

Eventually, we found the train. Getting home was easy — overhead rattler to London Bridge, down the escalator to the Northern Line, straight to Archway.

But before we reached New Cross station, the train stopped and sat there. The fans were dead Silent.

Then the shouting started.

"STAY TOGETHER! DON'T RUN! STAND!"

West Ham lads were barking orders. We were thinking — what the fuck is going on?

The train pulled into the station. And then — **BOSCH** — it kicked off.

"MILLWALL! MILLWALL!"

The train got hit with everything. Blind panic. In our carriage, a tall, skinny Black bloke — clearly a leader — took charge. The old trains had doors that opened from the outside, but he wasn't waiting. He leaned out the window, popped the door, and started swinging.

"COME ON YOU CUNTS! COME ON!"

He was kicking and punching any Millwall fan who came near. Other West Ham lads joined in — lashing out, trying not to get dragged off and swallowed by the mob.

It was bedlam. It felt like hours. Probably just minutes.

The train started to pull away. Doors slammed shut. Everyone checked themselves — bumps, grazes, bruises. But they were all there.

Jubilation. West Ham started singing. Back to the buzz. Back to the banter.

Next stop: London Bridge. We were out of the violence. It was home time.

So, we thought.

"London Bridge" came over the Tannoy. The train emptied. But Millwall were waiting.

As we walked toward the underground, we saw them — a proper mob. Hard faces. Big turnout. Scary looking geezers, these were men, not youngens.

West Ham seemed ready. They stayed on the platform. Mobbed up.

We knew what was coming. We walked past the Millwall lot, trying not to look. Got to the top of the escalator — and then the roar went up.

West Ham and Millwall had a field day.

Fists. Boots. Blood. It was war.

And then the news came. A young Millwall fan — just 18 years old — had lost his life at New Cross station that night.

A lad who came for football. Who never made it home.

RIP.

Chapter 7: Guerra De La Malvinas

The 2nd of April, 1982. Argentina decided the Falkland Islands were theirs for the taking. No warning. No diplomacy. Just a full-scale invasion.

Our Prime Minister at the time was Margaret Thatcher — Maggie. And Maggie wasn't having it.

She didn't flinch. She didn't hesitate. She sent a fleet of warships steaming down to the South Atlantic to take back what was ours and keep the Union Jack flying. It was the first time Britain had been called to arms since the Korean War ended in 1953.

As with everything in life — you don't let anyone take the piss. You don't let them take what's yours. And if they're bigger, louder, or more of them — you stand taller, shout louder, and hit harder.

Maggie wasn't called the Iron Lady for nothing. She made the call and we answered.

After 74 days of fierce fighting — in freezing seas, on bleak islands, with young lads dying far from home — the British forces retook the Falklands. General Leopoldo Galtieri surrendered. The Argentinian flag came down. Ours went back up.

But while the war raged thousands of miles away, it was felt right here — in the terraces, in the pubs, in the streets.

Tottenham Hotspur had two Argentinian stars in their side: Osvaldo Ardiles and Ricky Villa. They were magic on the pitch — they helped Spurs to an FA Cup Final. But war changes everything.

Villa didn't play in the final. Ardiles was out of the country and couldn't get back in. The mood had shifted. The country was at war. And suddenly, even footballers weren't immune.

I was 12 when those two joined Spurs. I remember it clear as day — I had a badge, light blue and white, that read: **"You can stick your Argentinians up your arse. Sideways."**

Tottenham were becoming the enemy early for me. And the war only sharpened that edge.

Fast forward to the FA Cup Final replay — Thursday night under the lights. The first match had ended 0–0. My two scoundrel pals — the same pair who held me while George L booted my shins at Hargrave Park — were going. No tickets, of course. But that never stopped them. And if you were with them, it didn't stop you either.

We made our way to Wembley. No drama on the journey. No stories worth telling. But the tension in the air? You could cut it with a Stanley blade.

It was a London derby — Spurs vs QPR. And I knew full well what Tottenham were capable of off the pitch. QPR didn't have the numbers, but they had heart. Gameness. They were tidy. And they were up for it.

What was strange — and I've never understood it — was how many of the Spurs mob came from West London. You'd think they'd be QPR. But no. They were Spurs. And they were hunting.

We followed them. Wembley Way. Under the flyover. And then — boom — they found each other.

Two proper mobs. No real old bill in sight. And it went off.

Punches. Kicks. The odd Stanley flashing in the chaos. You always had someone with a blade. Some clubs were known for it. Some scouse lads from Liverpool carried two blades with a matchstick wedged between — made the slice harder to stitch. Others dipped theirs in ammonia. True or not, it was terrifying to think how far people would go.

We were up on the stairs watching. My two pals were off — straight down, running with the Spurs lot. I stayed put. Neutral observer. Arsenal lad. But I'll say this — QPR gave a good account of themselves.

The QPR mob were very impressive.

Then came the cavalry. Kozzers on horseback, swinging long sticks like medieval knights. Clumping anyone they could reach.

The noise was unreal. Roaring. Screaming. Cars trying to leave the car park, horns blaring like that would stop the madness. Sirens. Hooves. Chaos.

I never found the two scoundrels again. They got swallowed up in the commotion. So, I started the walk-up Wembley Way, heading for the station. Baker Street was always lively — no matter who was playing.

By now I was 16. No longer a kid. No longer protected by the forcefield of youth. I looked like every other young lad out there — and that meant I was fair game.

That night, I realised something. When you're with your pals, going to dangerous games, it's all a laugh. You don't feel fear — just excitement. But when you're alone? That's when it hits you.

I didn't know who was who. Didn't matter. I was Arsenal anyway.

There was a scuffle on the platform. The first tube came in — half the platform emptied. I hung back. Waited for the next one. Luckily, it was the fast train — fewer stops, and the people around me looked like normal fans.

I got home in one piece. But something had shifted.

The war might've been in the South Atlantic. But the battles were happening here too — under flyovers, on platforms, in the shadows of stadiums.

And I was right in the middle of it.

A special dedication for a special friend from the Arsenal.

Mr Dale Hillier who fought for his country in the Falklands while the rest of us were running around at football, he actually fought in a war and now runs The Veteran Hotel and public house in Ryde on the Isle of White.

Lest we forget.

Chapter 8: Runaway

The Arsenal hadn't done much since Leeds beat us in the '72 Cup Final. The seventies were lean. But the tide was turning. In '78, we reached the FA Cup Final again — this time against Bobby Robson's Ipswich. Their first ever final. We were favourites. Hot favourites. This was supposed to be our fifth FA Cup win. Easy peas.

I've no idea why I didn't go to Wembley that day. But I was home, and Cup Final Day was sacred. The Girdlestone estate was decked out in red and white — scarves and flags hanging from windows like bunting at a royal wedding.

BBC coverage started at 11:30am. Interviews with players, Bob Wilson — our double-winning keeper turned pundit — chatting with John Motson. Then came the "Road to Wembley" montage. Goals, drama, glory. I was buzzing. Crisps, Mars bars, cola cubes — the full spread. I couldn't wait for 3pm.

They rolled out FA Cup Mastermind. Arsenal and Ipswich superfans answering questions only the obsessed could know. Then came the managers' interviews. I was ready to pop. Still two hours to go.

Team coaches left their hotels. Goal of the season aired. Then "Inside Wembley" — the changing rooms, the kits, the pitch. The tension was unbearable. The Band of the Guard marched out. "Abide With Me" played. The crowd sang. Half the stadium blue, half red and yellow. Flags waving. Roars rising.

And then — nothing.

Roger Osborne scored the only goal. Ipswich won. I sulked like a brat. Two Mars bars, a quarter of cola cubes, two litres of Coke — and a mood darker than the Thames. Losing to a poxy second division team.

But the next year came quickly. Arsenal was back in the final. This time against Manchester United.

We'd played Sheffield Wednesday four times in the cup run one game in freezing conditions, volunteers clearing snow off the pitch. Typical Arsenal. Never the easy route.

United were the media darlings. Biggest following in England. Could we beat them? Doubtful.

The estate was red and white again. But no Mars bars this time they were bad luck. I'd moved on to lemon Sherberts.

The game kicked off. Back and forth. Then — bang — Brian Talbot scored. We went wild. Talbot had played for Ipswich the year before. Lucky omen.

Then Frank Stapleton made it 2–0. Dreamland. Running around the house like a lunatic.

Half-time. We were cruising. Five minutes left. Easy.

Then Gordon McQueen scored. 2–1. Then Sammy McIlroy equalised. 2–2.

WHAT THE FUCK IS GOING ON?

I was too old to cry — but I wanted to. Wembley was rocking. United fans singing. Arsenal fans gutted.

Then came the moment.

Stapleton chested it to Brady. Brady ran. Outside of the left foot — slides it to Graham Rix. Rix whips it in. Ball drops over Gary Bailey's head. Alan Sunderland slides in…

GOAAAAAAAAAAL!

YES. YES. ARSENAL. The stadium erupted. The estate erupted. Our maisonette erupted.

We did it. We won the Cup. I loved my club. I loved being Arsenal.

By now, I was proper Arsenal.

Working Saturdays and school holidays at the firm where my dad worked.

I could afford home games. Some away games. Missed a few Saturdays — didn't want to let my dad down. He'd asked for the job for me. I had to be reliable.

Then came May 10th, 1980. Another Cup Final. Another second division team — West Ham. We were flying high. Four days later, we were playing Valencia in the European Cup Winners' Cup Final.

We wouldn't make the same mistake as Ipswich. Yes, we would. Lost again. Three finals in three years. Two lost to second division sides.

The highlight? Seventeen-year-old Paul Allen — youngest player ever in a Cup Final — clean through on goal. Just the keeper to beat. 100,000 watching. Live TV. Dream moment.

Then — **CRUNCH**.

Willie Young — big ginger Glaswegian — chopped him down like a redwood. Allen hit the turf face-first. Dream shattered.

Young patted him on the head. Shrugged at the ref. yellow card. West Ham fans raging.

The '79–80 season was the first time I really clocked the European games. Arsenal was in the Cup Winners' Cup. And we made the final — against Valencia. They had Mario Kempes. We had grit.

The final was in Brussels — Heysel Stadium. That had to be worth a trip.

I was working. Got myself a 72-hour passport from the post office. No one knew. Jumped on a ferry. Before I knew it — I was in Brussels.

Trouble outside the ground. Old bill heavy-handed. Dogs. Horses. Water cannons. They were expecting war.

Some of ours got nicked before the game. “Your friend is bye-bye,” the copper said. “He goes back to England.”

Inside, the fencing was crap. Ground run-down. Spanish fans firing flares at us. One geezer banging a bass drum non-stop.

Atmosphere? Electric.

Valencia was cocky. They’d beaten Barcelona. But we’d beaten Juventus — in Turin.

And that trip? That was violent. Proper violent.

But Brussels was something else. I was a kid. In a foreign country. No parents. No backup. Just me, my passport, and my club.

And I wouldn’t have traded it for anything.

The following account comes from one of Juventus’ main lads, reflecting on their clash with Arsenal in the 1980 Cup Winners’ Cup. It’s raw, honest, and shows how English fans were viewed across Europe at the time — admired, feared, and misunderstood. His words offer a rare glimpse into how the terraces looked from the other side of the divide…

Back in 1980 Juventus reached the semifinals in the old Cup Winners Cup and the opposition were Arsenal. Players and club alike were looking forward to reaching the final to be played in Brussels in the Heysel stadium, a ground that at the time had not achieved the bad name it would earn itself only 5 years later. Our main group was called Fighters, an English name, which should not surprise anyone as back then there was hardly anyone in Turin, in Italy or I dare say anywhere in Europe who did not look up to the English fans. I am not saying we liked them, just that we admired their unconditional support, their antics and their frequent riots. We had our style, the Ultras were no mugs, but let's be honest, the English boys had that little bit extra. Wherever they played, thousands of fans would turn up, drink the place dry and take on any comers. We were not too bad on our home turf, but away we were still miles away. The big names in England were rumoured to be MUFC, Chelsea, West Ham or Millwall. Arsenal was in theory not top dogs. That said they were English and Londoners and that seemed to qualify them as a worthy opponent.

It has to be stated that back then there was little information about what was happening in other countries and the little we knew was thanks to word of mouth and rumour. We had no previous experience with the Gunners, but them being English was enough for us. We were mostly still teenagers and relatively inexperienced, of course we had our battles in Italy, mainly with our city rivals from Torino, Fiorentina, Genoa and both clubs from Milan but on the international front we had a lot to learn and we believed Arsenal were the perfect test for us. From our slightly naive point of view, we thought we could match them, a few drunken English boys could not put up much of a fight, could they? We were proven wrong that night, we misread them, we didn't take them seriously and we had to eat humble pie. It's not that we didn’t try but with hindsight two aspects played against us. First and foremost, the fact that while we were mostly kids Arsenal had some grown men ready to fight.

When you are 19 and your opponent is 30 that makes a big difference. Secondly, in Italy when we took on a rival gang many battles did not end up in a proper toe-to-toe, as the weaker side (or the one that lost its bottle) ended up being run, and only the slowest got a hiding. More than once that night did, we attack small pockets of Arsenal, we usually outnumbered them but instead of doing one they just stood their ground. That was something we were not ready for, we hesitated, they didn't. There is little else to say. We bit off more than we could chew. Arsenal might have been a bunch of pissed fans, but they fought whatever the odds. On the odd occasion some smaller groups got ambushed and done but looking back that is not something to be especially proud of. Times were different, so much is true, and they did not mind either taking scalps of anyone they came across. One final consideration is required.

Back then we did not really know who was who, any English fan was seen as a legitimate target. Probably a large share of English fans was into fighting, though not all. We just attacked anyone, largely not being able to tell the difference between a proper lad and a drunken lout. Only a few months later in our stadium England got beaten by Belgium in the semis of the European Championship and trouble erupted again. I don't know if Arsenal were involved, I guess so but who knows. Out on the streets we wanted to have another pop at the English, but it was a bit of a repeat of the Juve-Arsenal affair. We only had a chance if we heavily outnumbered them. They deserved my respect and admiration for it. What I had no respect for was that inside the ground they attacked normal Italian fans who wanted no trouble. There are plenty of pictures where you can see dozens of English fans attacking a lone Italian wearing a suit, and even an old man in his late 50s. Totally out of order. I don't want to blame anyone, all the events are 45 years old and as I said before, times were different. After that double confrontation with Arsenal and England we understood we were not as good as we thought we were.

In Italy we were labelled as 'rabbits' nobody liked us but that was clearly rubbish. In Europe we had to learn our lessons and in the 1983/84 season we played the Mancs. It was a good day, but the Mancs were a tough bunch. And just one year later we played the Scousers in the Heysel tragedy. By that time, we knew the English well enough and were ready. Before the game our mob came across some Reds in the underground and it kicked off, one of them got slashed, some others got a pasting. There were more little skirmishes out on the streets before the tragedy unfolded. What happened inside is well known. It was a combination of poor policing and disastrous ticket allocation. Once more the tough English attacked innocent spectators. Basically, all the fans in the Z sector were dads with their kids, regular guys. A disgrace!! The English were only partially responsible, but they did charge into a sector full of normal fans. We charged across the pitch and goaded the scousers, to no avail. I guess they were too shocked about what they had done. The little respect I had for the English fans died on that fateful 29 of May 1985 in Brussels. As for Arsenal, they were our first English rivals in the 80's (not including Celtic in the same season). Arsenal was good and there is no more to be said.

Chapter 9: If Anyone Runs

I was five weeks short of my sixteenth birthday when I saw it the worst violence I'd ever witnessed in my journey into football hooliganism. And I'd seen plenty. But this? This was different. This was the day the Gooners came of age.

At fifteen, you think you're invincible. You've got a bit of fluff on your bollocks and a chip on your shoulder. You walk like you've earned your stripes, even if you haven't. We were the Young'uns — loud, proud, and fearless. We didn't know what we didn't know. And that made us dangerous.

Word was out: the Inter City Firm — West Ham's infamous ICF — were coming to Highbury. Not just for the match. They were coming to take the North Bank.

Now the North Bank wasn't just a terrace. It was sacred ground. Covered end. Home of the singers, the die-hards, the proper Arsenal men. Not lads chasing scraps — blokes who'd defend their patch like lions. It held 12,500 bodies on a match day, and every one of them knew what that end meant.

Taking an end wasn't just about numbers. It was about pride. You had to get deep into the stand, hold your ground, and survive the aftermath. If the old bill dragged you out and marched you to the away end, you'd get a hero's welcome — like you'd just come back from the beaches of Normandy.

And fair play — if 200 or 300 nutters stormed a stand that size, they were outnumbered ten to one. So, when they made it back to their own, they were clapped like soldiers.

But not today.

May 1982. We knew they were coming. We'd heard the whispers. ICF and they're Under 5s — the younger lot — were planning to take the North Bank. Most London firms had tried it. Some had succeeded. But not today.

Then the old bill steamed in — batons out, faces twisted. Chaos erupted. Smoke bomb went off. What the fuck? A smoke bomb? Cunts. Who did they think they were?

Normal fans fled onto the pitch and we had more room to move. More room to fight.

The ICF thought they'd done it. Thought the smoke and confusion meant victory. But as the fog cleared, we steamed into them again. From all angles. Punches flying. Adidas and Diadora alike landing. Bodies crashing.

It was relentless. The rush was unreal. Nothing — and I mean nothing — compares to that feeling. Adrenaline. Pride. Brotherhood.

The fight went on and on. Minutes felt like hours. And when a fight lasts more than a couple of minutes, it's serious. It's war.

Eventually, the old bill took control. But even they looked rattled. Shocked by the aggression. By the unity. By the sheer fucking will of the young Arsenal thugs.

We weren't just nippers anymore. We were the next generation. And we showed them how far we'd go. We tried to break through the police lines — desperate to finish it. To humiliate the firm that claimed to be the best in London.

In my opinion, they were happy to be behind the old bill. Giving it large, but glad for the protection.

That day, the Gooners came of age. And I was proud. Proud to be Arsenal.

After the game, things got messy. Me and a few of the lads got split up. We walked out of the North Bank — one of the boys said, "Blackstock Road or Finsbury Park?" We chose Finsbury. Big mistake.

Turned the corner. Felt the air change. Looked behind us — mob of older geezers. Proper men. Hard faces. Bad intentions.

"Who you looking at, you little cunt?" **BANG.**

Boot right up my arse. Hit my coccyx. Felt like a red-hot poker had been jammed up my arsehole. How I didn't scream, I'll never know.

We turned to front it out. Took a clump each. Kept walking. Another boot. More abuse. Proper mugging us off.

We got near Finsbury Park tube. Turned left onto Seven Sisters Road — no point heading to the station and getting battered again.

Down towards the Rainbow. Few Arsenal faces appeared. Then West Ham came from everywhere.

Toe-to-toe again. Me and a good pal ended up getting run down the road. Took a right opposite the Rainbow — onto a housing estate.

I picked up a half house brick. Protection. Seven or eight West Ham ran round the corner with us. No idea why. Maybe they were confused. Maybe Arsenal was behind them.

Didn't matter. New skirmish. I clumped one of their lads with the brick. Dropped it straight away.

He went down like a sack of shit. Out cold.

To this day, my pal says it was the hardest punch he's ever seen. If he reads this, he'll know — I hit the bloke with the brick. It was the only way to stop the onslaught.

Later we found out — while we were running around Finsbury Park, a good man called John Dickinson was stabbed to death by West Ham.

Cowardly. Senseless. Tragic.

RIP JD.

That day wasn't just a fight. It was a turning point. A line in the sand. We weren't just kids chasing buzz and bravado — we were Arsenal, and we stood our ground. We faced down one of the most feared firms in London and didn't flinch. We took punches, gave them back, and earned respect the hard way. But it came at a cost. Blood spilled. A good man lost. And the rush that once felt like glory now carried a shadow.

The following season West hams ICF Under 5s were in the west lower, they came nowhere near the north bank, they knew.

It would never happen again, you come in the north bank, and you will get kicked the fuck out of it.

They spent a lot of time the other side of the fence telling us what they were going to do to us and arranged that as the game finished, we would hit them head on at the bottom of the north bank stairs.

We weren't having it. We made the call —, get set, hold the line.

I remember it like it was yesterday. Standing at the top of the stairs, looking down at the entrance. And there they were. A tidy mob of geezers — flash clobber, swagger in their step, full of confidence. Led by a big black fella, laughing, goading, looking at us like we were nothing. They thought it would be easy. They thought we'd fold.

Some of us were nervous. You could see it in the eyes — lads who'd never been in a proper toe-to-toe. But then one of our Hackney boys stepped forward and barked it out:

"IF ANYONE RUNS, I'LL FUCKING CUT 'EM."

It wasn't a threat. It was law. You didn't run. Not today. Not ever. Better to take a hiding from the ICF than be marked by your own and never show your face again over the Arsenal.

They came up the stairs. And we met them head-on.

No hesitation. No backing off. Just fists, boots, and fury.

We smashed into them — proper toe-to-toe. They didn't expect it. They were backing off in no time.

We drove them down the stairs. Roaring. Buzzing. Proud.

But they regrouped. Came back up. Another go. Another clash.

And again — we held firm. Sent them packing.

The famous ICF were getting hammered. And I mean properly fucking hammered. They'll deny it to this day. But we know. We were there.

Chapter 10: I Met Stanley

I had this Valentino top — white, with a purple collar, a yellow patch on one elbow, a red patch on the other, and a cracking V crest right where your heart is. It was loud. It was proud. It was me.

Nice sunny day. We were playing Liverpool. We went in with them, and as the teams were coming out, **SHE WORE** went up — and it all went off.

Benetton shirts everywhere. You could tell we were Arsenal — we already had the green ones. But not me. Silly bollocks wore the stand-out Valentino to show the northerners how to dress. I looked like a walking target — but a stylish one.

The brawl went on for a while — great fun had by all. The Walrus (our mad copper) and his little firm got us back to the other side of the fencing. We started chatting with their lot — agreed to leave a bit earlier. The streets were where it was going to be.

We finally caught up with them at the top of Blackstock Road. It went backwards and forwards — proper running battles. Punches flying, lads slipping on paving stones, traffic swerving, objects being launched from all angles. Bottles, cans, even a fucking shoe at one point. Neither side getting real advantage — until one last push from us and they were off. On their toes. Gone. Vanished into thin air like smoke.

By now we were at Highbury Corner. This copper grabbed my face and said, "Where do you live?" Then **bang** — smashed my head against the Barclays bank door outside Highbury & Islington station.

I told him, "Archway." He said, "I've seen you in the thick of it three times today. Do yourself a favour — get on that bus and fuck off home. Otherwise, I'll nick you."

I took his advice. Got on the bus with a few pals. We got to Archway — top of Holloway Road, the A1 North.

We walked past the Kentucky. There were a few recognisable faces inside. I said to Clive S (RIP), "There's — those Scousers we had it with earlier."

No questions asked. We were in the Kentucky knocking the fuck out of everyone. Chicken chips airborne, ketchup bottles used as missiles.

Little did we know — they weren't just in the Kentucky. They were in the chippy and the Wimpy.

We'd bitten off way more than we could chew and knowing the manor — we made a tactical retreat.

Went home. Showered. Thought that was the end of it.

Roughly 8pm that Saturday evening, I was standing on the corner waiting for a pal. He saw me from a distance and screamed:

"AL — RUNNNNNNNN!"

I wondered what the fuck he was on about. Then I saw it.

A minibus pulled up beside me. Doors flew open. Scousers pouring out like it was a clown car at the circus — only these clowns were armed and angry.

I legged it onto the estate — straight to my sister's flat. She was down my mum and dad's caravan. And there I was — in my highly noticeable, give-it-large Valentino top. Smart as fuck. Surrounded.

They got me. I was beaten and trampled on so badly that the last words I heard were:

"You're dead now, cockney."

Then I blacked out. Pissed myself. Doctors said passing out probably saved my life — stopped them kicking me to death.

But that wasn't enough.

One of them came back. Pulled out a Stanley. Cut my legs.

I can never remember if it was 44 or 48 stitches. Doesn't matter. I was in a bad way. Brain swollen. Left-hand side looked like a giant purple love bite.

All because of that fucking Valentino top. And Arsenal being the best dressed in the country.

The stitches I could live with but to this day I have an arthritic neck and bad headaches because of the damage that I took.

Chapter 11: Unexpected Arrival

This football malarkey was becoming my life. Weekends weren't about rest — they were about movement, noise, adrenaline. There were adventures to be had, some good, some bad, and some that left a mark you'd carry forever.

I've never been one for reading football hooligan books. Too many supermen in diamond Pringles jumpers, all claiming they never ran, never backed off, always knew the exact numbers they were up against. It's bollocks. I've read a couple — one was decent, but halfway through another I had to put it down. Embarrassed for the bloke. Angry at the nonsense. Never picked one up again.

He was clearly superman.

But man — did I run fast at this particular game.

I can't even remember if it was a night match or just a grim Saturday evening. A few of us met outside Archway tube and made our way down to St Pancras for the short trip to Luton.

Luton was always a decent trip — close to London, easy to get back and hover between Kings Cross and Euston. There was always something bubbling around the stations, but that's a story for another time.

We arrived in Luton and unexpectedly, there was no welcoming committee. No youngens watching us from corners. No cheeky ambush. Just the usual piss-taking and banter on the train. I was always loud as an adult, but back then I kept quiet. Blended into the background. Never a face, never a name — but I was there, and plenty know I played my part.

The game itself was uneventful. We did what we always did — clocked who was about, nodded at the familiar faces, exchanged the usual "alright mate" without ever knowing names.

You'd see blokes so often you wouldn't dare ask who they were — it'd feel muggy.

I was about 15 or 16. Still figuring out where I stood in all this.

After the match, we moved out in a loose pack. Then came the noise — distant at first, then closer. Someone pointed down an alleyway. We followed. Big mistake.

Bricks. Bottles. Chaos.

When bottles start smashing around you, it's terrifying. You think you're next. They rarely shatter in a crowd, but when they do — they open you up or knock you clean out. It was proper scary. I remember thinking, "What the fuck am I doing with my weekends?" Surely there's something better than this?

We scrambled out of the alley. A few of ours had taken hits. There was a scuffle, but to our surprise, the Luton mob backed off. Some of our lads chased them down another alley that led to an open field — that's where one of ours got cut. Later, a Gooner from Luton helped sort a bit of revenge, but that's not my story to tell.

Luton's a strange gaff. Feels more northern than southern — rows of terraced houses, narrow roads, tight corners. There was a weird air about the place that day. We soon found out why.

We turned a corner and there they were — a mob of black lads, maybe twenty yards up the road, tucked just out of sight. We didn't know whether to go left or right. From memory, we went right. They were on our left. Now behind us.

Then came the roar.

Not a cheer. Not a shout. A roar. A primal, guttural sound — pure intimidation. It's the sound of aggression, of men ready to go. And weirdly, it gives you confidence. You hear that roar and you know it's on. You're not alone.

When the roar dies down, the fighting starts. It all happens in seconds.

They came at us. Toe-to-toe. Pushing, shoving, mad kung-fu kicks, punches flying. The main rule — don't go down. Never hit the deck. Because some mobs won't notice. Others will stamp you into the pavement.

Then, from behind a stopped bus, the white mob appeared. Now it was proper on top. Our numbers were thinning. Time for a tactical retreat — call it what you want, but it was time to run.

I was always a lumpy kid. Not built for speed. The kind of lad who got stuck in goal when you played footie with your mates. Maybe that's why I seemed brave — easier to fight than run and get caught.

My brother's eight years older than me. His best mate growing up was Martin C — another Archway boy. Big bloke. Gentle soul. Lost him to cancer in his early sixties — far too young. He has a younger brother, a proper terrace legend. Arsenal was in their blood.

People used to confuse them — same nickname, same aura. But on this day, it was the older brother beside me. We were at the back of the Herd, running like mad, being chased by a frenzied mob. We were at the back because we'd been at the front — doing the work. That's how it goes. Front line becomes rear guard.

Blokes were sprinting past us, shouting "STAND! Don't run from these cunts!" While they were running. Odd, that. Noise? Bravado? Fear?

The abuse from behind was getting louder. Closer. They were breathing down my neck. I was scared. Proper scared.

We passed a bus stop. The area got busier — shops, locals, confusion. Then I felt a hand grab my arm. I thought, "Fuck, no." But it was Martin. He had me moving so fast I could've challenged Carl Lewis.

To this day, I've no idea how far we ran. Or how long it lasted. But by the time we reached the station, the roar was going up again — everywhere.

Back at the station — bosh — I landed a cracker on one of their advancing lads. Wild punches. Quality kicks. I'd been doing karate since I was twelve, and it showed.

People were running around cars. Siren's blaring. Mayhem.

From what I saw, we got the better of Luton at the station. And from what I heard; the lads we got split from had some results too.

The station was ours.

Luton had organised well — the ambush on the corner was sharp. They had a good result. But we held our own.

The train back was buzzing. Bruises. Ripped clothes. Laughter. Adrenaline like you wouldn't believe. It's a feeling you can't replicate. Outside of this world, nothing comes close.

But he night wasn't over. We were only an hour from St Pancras. Was anyone waiting for us?

Thinking back, we had some mad times in Luton during the early to mid '80s. One incident stands out — sounds made up, but it happened.

Imagine being packed into a football ground. You've already clashed with the locals. You're pumped — that buzz only a hooligan understands. Better than any drug.

Then you hear it. See it. Commotion. People shouting, "It's West Ham! It's the ICF!"

In our end. How the fuck are they here? Why are they here? Who cares — this is our lucky day.

Chaos. Unfiltered. Unrelenting.

Fists and boots flying — not actual boots, mind. Gazelles. Sambas. Trims. Diodora's. Hair pulled. Clothes ripped. Dragging the opposition in with us.

It's a BUZZZZZZ.

It turned out that the train taking West Ham up to Birmingham had broken down at Luton.

Bedfordshire police must've had their hands full separating three warring mobs. Then the British Transport Police had to deal with us all getting back to St Pancras. And the rest of the night was spent scuffling through the backstreets of North London.

I've got great memories of Luton. But I can't write everything event down as this book has a purpose outside of the battles fought while growing up.

Chapter 12: Aunty Joan

The rivalry between us and the Mancs was getting more and more intense. We were becoming more respected by other mobs — they knew we'd be at Euston waiting for them before the game and definitely after. Tube stations were great for ambushes. We played them in the FA Cup semi-final that same season.

So far, we'd had some good run-ins. Now we had a semi-final at a neutral ground. Birmingham. Surely, we'd have fun up there — we were pretty even so far this season.

When they came to us in the league game, we didn't go to Euston. Instead, a few of us met at the Herbert Chapman — the boozer named after one of Arsenal's most successful managers. It sat on Holloway Road, just down from the tube station and across the road.

We were standing around, keeping our eyes peeled for spotters. Nothing. Quiet. Too quiet.

We were getting disappointed — convinced they'd be coming out of Holloway Road tube. Then, out of nowhere, a couple of youngens appeared under the railway bridge, pretending not to clock us. They stopped, turned, walked back.

A couple of our lads opposite the station came down and said, "They're outside the tube. Waiting. Letting their lot pile out so they can hit us full force."

From the Herbert Chapman, you can't see the entrance to Holloway tube. But we knew. They were coming. And they were in big numbers as always.

"There's fucking hundreds of 'em," one of ours said. "We've got our work cut out."

I wasn't running. Didn't care how many came out of that station. We were meeting them head-on.

Then it started.

UNITED! UNITED!

The acoustics under that bridge made it sound like the Royal Albert Hall. It echoed. It bounced. It roared.

And then they appeared.

Bouncing along the pavement like frenzied animals. Outnumbered? Mate — we were shockingly outnumbered. But I was with blokes I looked up to. Blokes I wanted to be like. I didn't care if they knew my name. I just wanted them to nod when they saw me. To know I'd stood my ground.

To this day, I'm not well known. But I did my bit. And I sleep well knowing this is my story.

Back to the Mancs — they started filling the other side of Holloway Road. For those who don't know it, it's a wide road. And they were filling it. Hundreds. No exaggeration. They always had numbers.

Then something happened — I don't know if it was planned or just perfect timing. Milk crates. Beer crates. From the pub. From the shops.

We ran at them like savages.

Traffic stopped. People sat in cars and buses, wondering what the fuck was going on. Praying nothing hit their windscreen.

Apparently, I had a crate in my left hand — swinging it like a maniac. I don't remember it. But I've been told I looked like a madman on speed.

The buzz was indescribable. Adrenaline. Fear. Glory.

Then the police horses came steaming out of Jackson Road. Hooves pounding. Old bill shouting. Two mobs going at it.

It was mesmerizing.

The frustrating thing with the Mancs was their size — their mob was so big, the old bill always turned up with them. They had spotters. So did the police. While they were gathering at Holloway tube, the cavalry was being called.

Back then, I swear the police let you go at it. They wanted it to kick off. So, they could wade in and smash you with truncheons. If they stopped it early, where was the fun for them?

We got backed off down Jackson Road towards Hornsey. The Mancs were pushed back to their meeting point and escorted to the ground.

Still, flying objects sailed over the old bill towards the Mancs. Not one nicking.

Those were the days.

Saturdays would involve going to football, going home, getting changed, and heading to the Whittington Stone or Brunswick to work out where we'd go that night.

Well, I got home and said, "Hello Mum."

"DON'T YOU FUCKING HELLO ME. YOU'RE A FUCKING EMBARRASSMENT."

What? What have I done?

My mind was racing. Had she found a dirty mag under the bed? Some gear stashed in the carpet in my cupboard. How could she? My head was spinning.

"YOU! YOU FUCKING—" Then my dad walks in. She shouts, "YOU FUCKING DEAL WITH HIM."

I'm lost. No clue what's going on.

My dad, calm as ever, sits at the kitchen table. "Been to football, son?"

"Yeah. You knew I was going. I always go Saturdays. You heard me talking to Barry and Gary at work."

Barry — my brother-in-law. Gary Turvey — top bloke, Arsenal through and through. We all loved the club. And I loved the off-pitch buzz just as much.

I sat down. Dad continued.

"Was there any trouble?"

Mum's still going off in the background — ashamed, embarrassed.

"No, Dad. Good atmosphere."

"No trouble at all?"

Now I'm panicking. Back then, you rented TVs. Got hire purchase from Jones Brothers. Had they been shopping? Seen something? Was it on the telly?

Dad, soft-spoken as ever: "So there was no fighting?"

"No, Dad."

"SO WHY THE FUCK WERE YOU RUNNING AROUND WITH A MILK CRATE THROWING BOTTLES AT PEOPLE?"

He was apoplectic. Screaming. I thought he was going to hit me — but his false teeth shifted, and I think that saved me.

Like a mug, I denied it. They weren't there. They didn't see.

Then Mum chimed in again.

"Do you know how embarrassed I am? Your Aunt Joan was on a bus in Holloway Road today. It got held up because two football gangs were attacking each other. And who did she see at the front?"

HER FUCKING NEPHEW.

I told you it came from a reliable source.

Chapter 13: Villa Park

The FA Cup semi-final against Man Utd was on played on the 16th of April 1983.

I was 17 years old and man, was I living for Saturdays.

What am I going to wear, this was a big deal.

We were proper casuals by this stage and we had to stay one step ahead of the northerners, how we dressed was important to us.

Decision made, faded jeans, Adidas Glorias (GLORIA GAYNORS= Trainers) Ball jumper with orange zip from next to Armpit.

I looked the absolute bollocks.

Tube down to Euston to meet up with the boys and the rattler to Birmingham.

We talk about bumping into the Cockney reds but really didn't need too as when we got to Euston, we jump on the escalator from the underground to the main concourse and as we are going up. We can see what were clearly West hams ICF were waiting at the top.

What a strange feeling going head on to some of what are now infamous book writers, well known and well respected.

We knew who they were straight away, what do we do, turn around and run down an escalator that is going upward to a certain battering.

Fuck that, the three of us as calm as anything got to the top and walked onto the concourse saying, ALRIGHT BOYS, just bluffed it.

These older gentlemen had no idea if we were West ham or Arsenal, us youngens all dressed similar, and they would have been looking for our faces.

We calmly made our way to the edge of this group as there were police everywhere and we said to one copper, we came up the wrong stairs mate, let us out of here they will kill us.

Luckily the copper let us out and a few of their lot realised and we exchanged pleasantries, like you West Ham mug and Gooner cunt etc.

They stated that they would get us later.

It turns out that they were on their way to Man city and we were off to Birmingham and the old bill really had their work cut out at Euston that day.

I bet half of the West ham didn't even go, they just wanted to get us at Euston, but they were on our manor, and in my opinion, we controlled Euston and the X.

During the game I remember seeing it go off down in the corner of the holt end where we were, but nothing worth writing about.

We lost again and our end emptied but we hung around and it was long before they arrived up our end, they came across the car park and up from the other end of the stadium and we clashed at the bottom of a grass hillside.

There were several clashes going on all over the place, the group that I was with were having fun with a group of mancs and they backed up against some hoarding for some building works that was being carried out. The hoarding went straight over and instead of going into the construction site we turned our attention to a scuffle that was taking place at the foot of the hill.

There were a few people getting grass stains on their faded Lois jeans on that day.

This went on for a while before the police could work out who was who and how to separate us.

The Birmingham police did not take any prisoners, they were as violent as any football fan.

Imagine getting paid overtime to have a tear up with no concerns about getting nicked and you are even allowed to use a weapon, they fucking loved it.

Thugs in uniforms.

Later on in life I went on to meet a policeman who was a Crystal Palace fan who was working as a Robo Cop when Millwall had a riot at home to Birmingham at the Den.

He was chatting away and his wife was telling us how worried she gets because on that day the Millwall bods were trying to pull him out of the police line and in with them and he has his shoulder dislocated, but when he spoke, it was with the same excitement, joy and passion of a hooligan. HE LOVED IT.

We walked the way the old bill had planned for the Arsenal fans, got pie n chips and made our way back to new street station, this was the Brumby equivalent of London's Euston.

On the way back to New Street, the whole platform was full of Arsenal and as defiant losing fans are, they were singing Arsenal songs and some were angrily waiting for the train to get us into town.

What was strange was that there seemed to be as many Arsenal fans on the other platform going the other way.

What we thought was our train coming in to the station at a snail's pace but it wasn't stopping, it was full of mancs banging on the windows and some of the rowdier barmies were banging on the windows from the outside, the train was obviously not going to stop but none the less it was rowdy, then the moment arrived that will live with me forever.

A loud mouthed manc was hanging out of the door window abusing people.

Somone pinged him, no matter how slow the train was going, to be hit while you are moving left the bloke hanging out of the door for a few second then he fell back into the train with everyone on our platform were laughing their heads off.

The bloke who threw the punch of a lifetime must have shattered his hand. Ouch.

When we got to new street and met up with the rest of ours, we all congregated in the station, a mob appeared from the other side of the station and we immediately knew that they were mancs, we were across the station in what seemed like seconds, I think that the reason that the mancs scattered down platforms and onto the tracks was purely because of the speed that we went at them.

There was no bravado, no sussing each other out, nothing but pure instant aggression.

We emptied the station of Mancs pretty rapid.

After that nothing much happened and some of made our way back to London, we were on a barmies (normal scarf wearing fans) train, we were just fucking about having a laugh and making fun of each other the barmies and as Birmingham isn't far from London, we were trying to work out where to have a drink.

The rattler pulls into Euston and we disembark and there they were.

West Ham waiting on the ramps for us.

They weren't looking for our barmies, they were looking for us, for Gooners, dressed like them, some of them knew our faces.

How the fuck are we getting out of this one.

This lot were like watching a National Geographic documentary about a pack of Wolves who are sitting on a hill looking down through a flock of sheep, while lick their lips at the thought of getting the juiciest ones.

Well, on this day, we were the juicy ones.

Never in my life have I tried to blend in so much with a load of barmies, I put my nut down and stared at my laces as best I could.

There was a bloke beside me singing about the Arsenal, wrapped in a flag and more scarves than I have ever seen one man wear.

He was oblivious of the awaiting slavering wolves on the ramp, so he should be that weren't looking for him, they wanted people like me.

I asked him for a scarf, NO was the reply, I begged him for a scarf, again, NO was the sharp reply.

I had to explain that the gentlemen on the ramp would beat me up and being a nice person, I would hate to have to nick one of his scarfs, regretfully, He wasn't very nice and I had to take one of his scarfs to blend in.

We managed to get through them, no drama, no clip around the ear hole, nothing and in amongst Arsenal fans who were singing, and credit to the West Ham boys, they knew who they wanted and never touched anyone.

When we got out of the tunnels under Euston we started to laugh and breath with a regular heart beat and we walked straight into one of their spotters outside the main set of doors.

All on his own, he looked around and suddenly we were there.

Hello Son, what are you up to.

He replied, nothing much, just waiting for my pals.

I said, cor they will have the needle, coming back from Birmingham after getting beat by Utd again.

This kid was now in a total state of confusion and as he now thought that we were west ham who were going to give him a clump for being Arsenal, to thinking that we were West ham and that he was safe.

So, he fessed up and told us that their lot had separated into three little firms and that there was no way the Gooners would get out of Euston without bumping into them.

He even told us that the Arsenal were getting too big for their boots, cheeky fucker, he did have a nice jumper on though, which was odd for west ham as we always though that they were never quite as well dressed us.

He was relieved of his jumper and the few quid that he had in his pocket, tube ticket etc.

He never took a clump and wasn't hurt in any way, I will tell what was hurt, this budding hooligan's pride.

He must have felt so angry, imagine having to explain to the ICF who were planning an ambush on the Arsenal that you were taxed while waiting outside Euston, by the people that you were waiting for.

When I was younger if that had happened to me, I had such a bastard temper, I would have been in tears of rage and probably have taken a whack.

This kid had to show his face to the men that he was out to impress, that would hurt more than any black eye and live with you.

We walked around a bit and kept our distance watching to see what would happen with each train's arrival.

There were no mobile phones in those days, so finding anyone would be potluck so we walked down to the X and jumped on the tube back to the Archway.

Chapter 14: Spud-U-Like

Man, you had a big mob, what a mob.

There were loads of them, even though I am firm believer that 80 goodness that know each other with good hearts is more than enough against anyone.

None the less, it doesn't matter what I think, there were loads of them, coming from all over the country, they had mobs within mobs. Probably all out to prove themselves to the main Manc mob.

We reached the semi-final of the league cup, this tournament has always had a two legged semis final system and we played them at home.

A dark horrible night, we knew that there would be a few of them that wouldn't get in and there would be little offs (fights) outside the ground during the game.

They meeting were often the best ones because sorted out the men from the boys, because they aften last longer as the old bill were in the ground and the coppers on horses were site outside the ground.

Remember that there were no mobile telephones, and a lot of hooligan clashes were as much about luck as they were about hunting them down, or indeed being hunted.

A few of us walked around the corner, down from Highbury fields along the Victorian houses where all the well-off people lived, beautiful streets, even when I was young I dreamed of living in one of those houses, we did a right from Highbury hill on to Aubert Park and got half way up the hill and over the top of the hill we see a fucking cracking mob taking up the whole road and maybe 30 ft in front was 5 of 6 of ours walking quickly, so we assumed that this mob in the distance was the Arsenal.

Within a split second, one of the group, a skinny Archway boy who lived in the block opposite me with a mop of blond hair shook his head and said ``Don't go up there Al, there fucking Mancs so as we joined the group coming down the hill, the Mancs realised that we were Arsenal and came down the hill at us, I can honestly tell you that I have no idea what happened to the others because I was knocked into a bush and fell through and landed at the bottom of a stair well of a basement flat of one of the houses that I loved so much.

The thought of that fall while I am sitting here typing this is making me cringe. It wasn't a little fall.

None the less I thought that I would just stay down the stairwell and recover for long enough to be able to stick my head out of the gate and regain an ounce of composure.

I made my way down to Drayton Park and met up with our main lot.

You could always find some of us down near the away coaches but against UTD, that didn't matter so much because there were probably as many from fucking Guildford as there was from Salford. There was now about 50 of us, (here we go, I am counting like the other books) this lot were proper, and, in all honesty, it will take a good mob to go through us.

We were now marching up to Holloway Road and you could not have wished for more, they were there, down the side street, maybe heading to our boozer, the favourite and we were behind them.

No police horse at that moment, even though they were in Drayton Park, the call goes up and we clash in the middle of the road. Shouting and hollering, clenched fists and kicks flying everywhere. It's not time before the police horses are racing down the street and doing their best to separate the warring mobs.

Was this a big fight, did it last ages, was there a winner? Who cares.

When you are in the middle of it, time and motion of others goes out of the window, and you never really know who amongst your lot was throwing punches or moving around strategically and looking like they were involved.

Sometimes it easy to tell who they were, because they spent the next two hours saying, did you see when I knocked this bloke out and that 6ft 5in bloke with the muscles went over like a sack of shit when I clumped him.

You must get those blokes everywhere, but they are good to have a round because the most important thing is that they don't actually run, they just don't really fight.

Now that takes skill.

There's not only 50 of us there would have been 100s somewhere else so they are either missing each other or battling out with the Mancs, when the old Bill separated us, we went out onto Holloway Road and then you could see it, the whole of Holloway Road was flashing with blue lights and police on horseback with hi visibility uniforms lighting up from the car lights sitting in the traffic.

What a spectacular sight.

We start to make our way down it what must look like someone trying to stop himself from shitting, because we didn't want to run to attract more police attention, but we wanted to walk as quick as we could.

When we got down there it was the clearly the end of a proper turn out between two mobs.

The following week, it our turn to go up there.

We meet at Euston; a few beers and we are ready to go.

Some bods would play cards, others were telling stories and taking the piss out of each other, some were off making fun of the southerners who were travelling up to support Man utd.

Although I despised the southern Utd and Liverpool fans because they were glory hunting tossers, I often felt sorry for their normal fans who had to sit on trains full of hooligans that were going up there to do battle with their enemies.

These fans were not getting bashed but verbally abused and on occasion, they would be mugged.

We get into Manchester late afternoon and hang around Piccadilly station but nothing is happening so we decided to get the train to old Trafford and this was the

funniest trip ever.

We had a mixed-race fella that came with us, a wild boy gap in the front of his mouth where a tooth was missing and he was on brilliant form chatting to the commuters.

He was going at them like a stand-up comedian, nothing rude or abusive, just fun, the commuters were even laughing.

Imagine sitting on the rattler going home from a days work and a group of loud young cockneys jump on.

All full of themselves with anticipation of beating the Mancs on and off the pitch.

On the pitch was highly unlikely, as we were already 4-2 down from the home game.

Who cares, we are the Arsenal.

I don't know why but we couldn't find any Mancs that partook in the same hobby as ours, we walked around the concourse and again not much happened, not anything

that stayed in my memory, so we made our way into the shit hole and as we got in, they must have turned up and our lot who were queuing up to get in the ground were going at it with them outside and us lot inside could not do anything.

They won and knocked us out of the cup.

Oh well, we need to get away from the old bill and find the Mancs or at least the cockney reds will get it at Piccadilly station.

Now I have a shady memory on this part as it was 41 years ago.

The old Bill either wrapped us up and made us wait on bit of waste ground before letting us go back to Piccadilly or when we left Manchester, we had to change, and the old Bill fucked us around somewhere else.

None the less, we were at Piccadilly station and there was a couple of little rare ups

but nothing special and the then a Datsun 260ZX was driving up the pavement trying to run Gooners over.

Apparently, it was one of the infamous leaders of one of the Manc mob, a black fella, well known to all.

Nothing was really happening, and we all went off to get food at any gaff that was still open.

I chose SPUD-U-LIKE, we were all queuing waiting for our food, know that the old bill had fucked us around just long enough for us to be put on a shit train home.

We all really needed to eat because of the nasty journey home that was in front of us, and this copper comes running in.

RIGHT GET OUT THE TRAINS HERE, screaming like a madman.

Fuck off I'm waiting for me food was the reply from one of ours at the counter, I was still nowhere near the counter, and I was Hank Marvin (starving).

The brave or as it turned out, stupid young policeman now made the mistake of his life.

He pulled out his stick and shouted GET OUT NOW, with the end part of the sentence being incredibly unprofessional, I say that part in jest.

His words WHICH ONE OF YOU COCKNEY BASTARDs WANTS IT FIRST, NOW

FUCKING GET OUT.

As the word OUT left his mouth, someone hit him with a piping hot jacket potato with melted cheese, straight in his face.

Man did that young policeman scream, he was in blind panic and to be fair, so was everyone who witnessed it.

It was actually horrible to see and you know that it must have hurt like a bitch and secondly, those northern old Bill are now really going to have the needle (angry) with us.

We then thrown on a night train back to Euston, this was what can only be described as a cattle train, it definitely wasn't a passenger train.

We sat where we could and arrived back at Euston at 04.45 in the morning and the

only people on the streets were the brasses who were trying to find their last punter of their shift and junkies.

I had to be in work at 07.30 so hung around the X (Kings Cross) until a café opened and got some breakfast.

Luckily, I worked in Brewery Road, opposite the Ville (Pentonville prison) its only along the Cally (Caledonian Road) so was in work on time that morning, man was I tired.

The rivalry between us and the Mancs was getting more and more intense as we were becoming more and more respected by other mobs, they knew that we would

be at Euston waiting for them before the game and definitely after the game, the tube stations were great for ambushes.

Chapter 15: The Pig & Whistle

To this day, I still can't remember whether we started our nightclub wars with Ladbroke Grove QPR before the infamous Pig & Whistle turn-out, or whether our attack on the boozer kicked it all off.

We met at the usual spot. Today's foe: QPR. A game mob. Not big in numbers — like when they faced Spurs at Wembley — and probably underestimated by the big firms, same way people still speak negatively about the Arsenal, but these boys could hold their own.

People forget — our grounds are in proper rough parts of London. A game boy is a game boy, no matter who he supports.

One of ours must've decided we'd get off the tube at Latimer Road. That meant a mile walk to Loftus Road — twenty minutes through enemy territory. Mobs did this to try and get at other mobs undetected. Always a risk. Because 150 lads walking both sides of the street — no matter how much you spread out — it's obvious. It's a mob.

The buzz on the tube was electric. I had no idea we were getting off at Latimer Road — hardly anyone did. Only the top boys knew what was coming.

As the tube pulled in, the shout went up: **"OFF! GET OFF!"**

We stepped off, assuming we'd march to the ground and hit QPR by surprise, dodging the old bill.

You do the usual look-around — make sure everyone's off of the tube and on the platform together.

Latimer Road's an old station, stairs leading down to the street, surrounded by housing estates. You're with pals, blokes you'll fight side by side with — even if you don't know their names. They're Gooners. That's all that matters.

You feel invincible. Like you could take on an army, but when you get off a tube, you've no idea where you'll land in relation to enemy fire. And we weren't told what station we were getting off at.

We casually walked down the stone steps — nearly out onto the street — and then **boom**.

Glass exploded around us. Bottles, pint glasses, ashtrays, pool balls — anything that could be thrown was coming our way. It was like stepping into a war zone. The air was thick with the sound of shattering glass and the thud of wood on bone. And then — I swear on my life — an old pram came flying through the air. A fucking pram. It spun above us like something out of a cartoon, wheels rattling, before crashing into the railings beside the stairs. That's when we knew — this wasn't just a few lads having a pop. This was an ambush.

Like the longbowmen at Agincourt, these fuckers were dug in and ready. They knew we were coming. They had bats, axes, lumps of wood, and a full arsenal (No pun intended) of household missiles. It was raining chaos.

Us lot at the front took the brunt. We were getting battered while the main bods behind us were still trying to get out of the station. We had nowhere to go — just had to stand firm and hope we didn't take a direct hit.

Outside the station was the Pig & Whistle — and it was like a scene from Football Factory on steroids. Glasses flying, fists swinging, bodies crashing into walls and bins. We ran at them. Met them head-on in the street. No hesitation.

It was hand-to-hand carnage. Everyone was fighting. No passengers. The QPR boys had help — local lads from the manor, probably not even football fans. Even the Rastafarians were launching bottles at us. I always thought Rastas were peace-loving, chilled-out blokes. Not these ones. These ones were raging.

We were proper going at it — punching, kicking, grabbing whatever we could find. Missiles that had been thrown at us were now being used as weapons. No one was backing off. It was raw, tribal, and relentless.

Two game mobs, toe-to-toe in the middle of a West London Street and then the sirens. Police vans came screaming down the road, tyres screeching, doors flying open. Blue lights flashing off broken glass and bloodied faces.

We later heard that most of QPR's main mob had already gone to the ground, but you always heard that sort of shit when you've had a bit of a result, so it didn't matter.

We'd had our fun and we did more than hold our own on their manor.

A couple of ours got nicked — which always ended in piss-taking. The old bill would leave the van doors open, scoop up a few bods, and chuck them in the back. We'd stand outside, taking the piss, knowing they'd be off to the magistrates to pay a fine.

We marched to the ground. Not much else happened.

The game itself? Memorable for one reason: Lee Chapman.

Lanky. Dog-shit player. Loftus Road had the only artificial pitch in the league — and Chapman couldn't get his head around it.

At the best of times, he looked like an epileptic giraffe. But that day? He was at his worst.

Every time the ball came near him, even we — the Arsenal fans — were laughing.

Most memorable moment? He jumped to head the ball after it bounced in front of him — either jumped too early or had already landed by the time the ball sailed over his head. Calamitous.

The game ended. Like always, we mobbed up for a walk of strength — giving it large on the opposing manor.

It kicked off quickly on the corner of the stand. Few punches thrown — nothing major. But for some reason, we split up. A few ended up at Shepherd's Bush — and we found them.

Scuffles were already breaking out on both sides of the road. No old bill anywhere. Just mad scrapping and people running around.

I went charging across the road at a few of their lads. Started going at it. At that stage of my life, I was doing kickboxing — probably looked quite impressive. Nothing like a few high kicks to scare the life out of people (even though the higher the kick, the less the power).

This carried on along the road heading towards Notting Hill station.

They had a little geezer with them — seemed to be listened to by most of their firm. Whatever he shouted, they adjusted to. Must've been one of their main lads.

We later found out his name — and sadly, he recently passed away. To this day, I don't know if he was Chelsea or QPR. I think he ran with both. Chelsea liked him. In later years, he was more connected to them. Maybe he was just having a day out with his QPR pals.

He respectfully attended the funeral of a friend of mine who passed away in October 2007. Turned up with some Chelsea bods — brought a Chelsea Head-hunters wreath.

During one of our midnight patrols down at Euston, we often bumped into QPR. They had a few good lads — a mixed-race bod who was as game as a stone, and so were his pals.

I remember one particular time — saw a scuffle in the distance at night.

It was funny as fuck. Early '80s — everyone was bodybuilding, taking steroids, boxing, doing kung fu. We'd go to late-night pictures down the Odeon in Holloway Road, come out in the early hours, and there'd be blokes pissing about re-enacting the moves they'd seen. I can't write the Chinese noises Bruce Lee made — you'll have to imagine them.

The scuffle between Euston and the X was maybe ten blokes having a tear-up. But the black and mixed-race ones looked like they were doing kung fu — reminded me of ninjas doing stealth attacks in a bad kung fu movie.

If we'd known who it was, we'd have run up there. But it could've been Spurs vs Millwall for all we knew — so we just watched.

As mentioned earlier, there was a real Archway (Arsenal) vs Ladbroke Grove (QPR) rivalry in nightclubs down the West End. It spread to Hackney Road, Bethnal Green Road with West Ham, Wood Green, and the Mayfair and Eltens in Tottenham.

Arsenal even ventured to Zero 6 in Southend — turned it over. West Ham weren't happy about that one.

The Lyceum was always fruity. You never knew what was going to happen. If you'd been active in there, you'd stay away for a couple of weeks — bouncers wouldn't let you in. But you'd still wait outside to pick off the West London lot.

The DJs didn't help. Every week they'd shout: "Anyone here from North London?" — we kept quiet. East London — nice roar. West London — nice roar. Then South London — sounded like a goal had been scored at Wembley. They were everywhere.

We had a few bods around Archway who loved a tear-up but weren't football people. They'd come out with us sometimes.

We had a ginger geezer with us one night — SD — a proper quality amateur boxer. Tough as nails. Even his sister could handle herself. One of those families where you just knew not to take liberties.

It all kicked off as usual. I was toe-to-toe with a Ladbroke Grove bod — giving it everything. Bear in mind, I'd boxed at primary school, had a stint at Alexandra Palace Boxing Club (didn't like it, didn't stay long), and by twelve I'd switched to karate. I was better with my legs than my fists, so I thought I could look after myself.

But this geezer wouldn't drop. I was throwing everything at him — punches, kicks, the lot. Then I felt a tap on my shoulder.

It was SD.

"Leave him, Al. Leave him."

I stepped back. And just like that — **PING**. One punch. The Ladbroke Grove lad slid down the wall like a tin of paint had been lobbed at it.

That's the difference between thinking you can fight — and really being able to fight.

One nice thing that came out of those days was a proper gent in the Arsenal mob — now a cabbie from West London. During one of the bigger Lyceum battles, the scrap spilled onto Charing Cross Road and up towards Trafalgar Square — where you could catch a night bus home.

The West London lot were hunting down any Arsenal they could find. My pal clocked the danger, jumped into a queue with a group of West London birds for cover — made it look like he'd been out with them all night.

They were total strangers. But that night in the early ’80s? He found more than safety.

He’s still married to one of them.

Chapter 16: Do You Really Want to Hurt Me

Three of our lot had 18th birthdays close together and decided to organise a disco riverboat party along the Thames a proper knees-up on the water.

The Archway crew met at the Whittington Stone for a few beers and a bit of bunny about the night's plans. We were sharp dressers — or so we thought. Jaeger jumpers, Farah round-the-houses with tailored slits so they sat perfectly over your college shoes from Ravels down Seven Sisters Road. My dogtooth Bow N Arras were the dogs' bollocks. We even went through a stage of wearing glasses with plain glass in them — what on earth were we thinking?

The boat party was for the older lot. I was probably 16 at the time, but none of that mattered. We thought we were geezers.

The party kicked off and the disco music was spot on — The Whispers, Shalamar, George Benson belting out across the river. Everyone was having a good time. Then we heard a fuss.

There was a truly great man we all looked up to — a black fella built like a bear. For some reason, he threw a bit of a wobbler. The only one strong enough to calm him down was another black lad we knew — a bodybuilder with a booming laugh and a sheepskin coat that made him look like a walking sofa. If you were the opposition and saw him coming, you'd start praying.

The boat party wrapped up around 1am. Someone said, "I wonder if anyone's up at the Lyceum or Busby's." By "anyone," they meant Spurs, Chelsea, QPR, Millwall, West Ham — the usual suspects. So yeah, "anyone" was the perfect word.

Off we trot — up the side of Embankment and Charing Cross stations, onto Charing Cross Road.

Busby's was a nightclub near Oxford Street. Just a doorway with a couple of old lump bouncers. If they let you in, you walked straight down mirrored stair risers into a decent little gaff. But if you were mob-handed, you could come unstuck — it wasn't far from Somers Town and Holborn, and they had plenty of handy bods who loved a late-night tear-up.

We got there just before kicking-out time and waited outside to see if any known faces appeared. The mouthy bouncers started asking why we were standing around and told us to fuck off. They should've kept their mouths shut. We were minding our own business, but now they were under pressure — we had lads with us who saw bouncers as a challenge, not a threat.

What saved them from getting smashed to bits was the club lights coming on. Time for the punters to leave.

Picture it — hundreds of people pouring out, and us milling around. No one could tell how many of us there were, or how many of the enemy might be lurking.

Then the little bloke from QPR/Chelsea — the one I mentioned earlier — came bowling out with a few bods. One of my pals, a ginger lad, said something to him. He gave it large. Next thing, it's about to go off and the geezer shouts:

"DO YOU KNOW WHO I AM?"

As he said it, both me and the ginger lad clumped him. Then we found out how many pals he had with him — and the answer was: not enough.

Scuffles broke out everywhere. When that happens, blokes with their non-football pals get involved — it's instinct. The bonus for us was that we all knew each other. The other groups were fighting blind and getting clumped from all directions.

We started walking home when a mob of half a dozen bods started singing Tottenham songs outside the Dominion.

It was like Christmas had come early.

It gets better.

Part of the journey home took us through Camden Town. There was a nightclub called Camden Palace — big old gaff on the bottom of Camden High Road, right on the edge of notorious Somers Town.

We walked past the Wimpy Burger place — still open — and strolled in like we owned it. The gaff was full of weirdos.

Makeup everywhere. Bold, outrageous clothing. Some of them you couldn't tell if they were male or female. It was like walking into a different planet.

Before you know it, one of my Archway pals was arguing with this big lump — towering over him. And believe me, this bod wasn't intimidated. My pal could fight, but you could see the confusion on his face.

Was he arguing with a big bird? Or a geezer dressed like a bird?

Either way, this thing wasn't backing down.

The situation calmed down and we left. Walking up the road, the banter kicked off.

"What the fuck was that?" "Ha ha — you didn't know whether to fuck it or fight it!"

We laughed about it for weeks in the pub.

Then came Thursday night. Top of the Pops.

This new group came on — Culture Club. And this bloke called Boy George started singing:

"Do You Really Want to Hurt Me..."

We all looked at each other.

Boy George was the Wimpy bloke.

Chapter 17: Micky Droy November '83

Micky Droy was a unit of a central defender who played for Chelsea for 15 years. For anyone older than 25 at the time of writing this, it was when Chelsea was shit — up and down like a whore's drawers. A nothing club on the pitch, but they always had a fearsome reputation off it.

Testimonial games were usually played at the end of the season, a thank-you for long service, with the money going to the player's pension fund. Bear in mind, players earned well back then — but not like the self-centred pricks of today.

This one was shoehorned into the regular season — a cold Tuesday night under the lights.

Arsenal was now a force to be reckoned with — off the pitch more than on it. The weekend before, we'd played away to Aston Villa in Birmingham. Always a good one.

You didn't have to leave Euston too early, so you could look for other mobs. And Birmingham's central station meant you could bump into all sorts. Villa themselves were formidable opponents — proper game lads.

Back then, trains and coaches were where all the planning happened — upcoming games, ambushes, who was turning out. And for the Villa trip, all the talk was about Chelsea on Tuesday night.

Why? Because apparently, one of Chelsea's superstars out of Streatham had been stabbed over on our manor — down the Caledonian Road — one Friday or Saturday night.

The Cally was rough. Not just council estates — it was the main artery from Kings Cross to Holloway Road, where the Arsenal lived.

My mum and her siblings were born down the Cally. Almost all my cousins grew up there. One estate in particular — Bemerton — produced some maniacs. One family went on to become one of the UK's biggest and most deadly crime syndicates.

The flats had 4- and 5-bedroom units, so they were getting all the big families from Somers Town, Angel, Camden, Kentish Town, and Archway. That estate saw shootings, petrol bombings, glassing's — and with football on the doorstep and the X (Kings Cross) nearby, it was as rough as fuck.

Back to the stabbing — one of the Herd from Archway had allegedly plunged this Chelsea bod. And there was talk of Chelsea wanting revenge. Even talk of them trying to grab my pal and pull him away from us.

Let's skip what happened at Villa — other than we beat them 2–6 — and the Midlands old bill were evil. If you stepped off a crowded pavement, they'd whack you with their sticks and they fucking hurt.

Excitement was building for Tuesday's trip to Chelsea. We met at the Arsenal Tavern on Blackstock Road. Proper turnout — better than we'd hoped for.

Everyone was buzzing. The excitement alone was addictive. There was only one person quieter than usual — and you could understand why.

He wasn't just quiet — he was carrying something heavy. You could see it in his eyes. That thousand-yard stare, like he was scanning every corner, every doorway, every face. He knew the whispers. He knew the rumours. Chelsea wanted blood — and his name was on the list.

It's one thing to front it out when you're just another face in the mob. It's another when you're the one they're coming for. Every step across London must've felt like walking into a trap. Every laugh around him probably sounded distant. He didn't flinch, didn't moan, didn't ask for protection — but you could feel the tension coming off him like heat.

We made sure he was never alone. Not for a second. Because if Chelsea wanted him, they'd have to go through all of us.

The shout went up. We herded up and left the boozer. I was amazed how many bods that pub could hold.

Straight down to Arsenal tube and across London on a weeknight at rush hour. We had to keep the mob together — no splitting up on this one.

Can't remember what station we got off at, but the journey was full of laughter, piss-taking, and — unfortunately — a few commuters lost items. All mobs had urchins who used the crowds to earn a few quid.

Another thing with mobs — you can leave a pub with 100 and arrive with 60. But not today. Our numbers held. No one was letting our pal down.

We marched to the ground from a direction Chelsea weren't expecting. Almost silent. Just before the forecourt of the Shed — that big rusty metal stand — there's a humpback bridge.

As we reached it, one of our overzealous youngsters shouted something like "EIE" or "Gooners!" All I heard was a smacking sound and "SHUT THE FUCK UP." I was right beside the bloke who gave the slap — game as a stone, still is.

We appeared at the top of the bridge and marched onto the forecourt. Chelsea got run everywhere.

The ones on the forecourt split — disappeared in all directions. We walked back out towards Fulham Broadway station, where the old bill was waiting. They sent horses up towards the Shed entrance — we were banging anyone who wanted it.

By the time we reached the North Stand, we'd gone through everything they had to offer.

Inside the ground, we were down behind the goal. A big mob appeared at the top of the North Stand — being escorted towards us. We knew they weren't Arsenal, but the police didn't.

As our overzealous youngster had shouted earlier, a few of theirs shouted "Chelsea!" Just a few feet from the fence line. That was enough.

Mayhem. Panicking policemen. If they hadn't shouted, they might've got in with us — and the old bill would've had no chance.

After the game, we herded up and were escorted to the station. The experienced among us knew what was coming.

An ambush.

Three reasons:

1. Too many of their firm had left the ground before full-time.
2. It was too quiet outside — no one waiting for us.
3. In my opinion, we'd taken the piss.

We squeezed onto a tube — desperate to make sure we were with our faces. And that our pal — the one Chelsea wanted — was on our carriage.

He was. And now he looked more relieved than earlier.

We pulled into (I think) Earls Court — and they were there. Crowded platform. The tube driver pulled up and Chelsea hit the train so hard before the doors opened, I thought it might roll over.

Then the doors opened — and the fighting started.

If you've never fought from inside a train against a mob on a platform — the idea is to do damage but not get pulled off. Or pulled on. Depends where you start.

It was chaos, but one memory will live with me forever.

One of our black lads from Balls Pond Road area grabbed a fluorescent light tube from inside the carriage — and stabbed it into the forehead of a Chelsea lad.

These tubes are thin glass, filled with powder. I'm not skilled enough to describe it properly — but imagine a Star Wars character sticking a lightsabre into someone's head. It didn't come out the other side — but it looked like it did. The tube shortened as it went in, giving the impression it was disappearing into his skull.

Probably didn't do much damage. But fuck me — it looked good.

The doors shut. The tube pulled away. And our man was still with us.

We stayed on guard for the next few stops. Later, a handful of us wandered around the X and Euston — but they didn't turn up.

A great evening had by all.

While we're on the subject — I was in the Mayfair nightclub a few years later with two girls off my estate. They knew a couple of birds, and one had a single bloke with her. He looked just about as nervous as me — being in a club on Tottenham High Road and not being Spurs.

We got talking. His first question: "Are you Spurs?"

I knew he wasn't — he looked uncomfortable. Whether he was telling the truth or not, he said he was D O'K from Streatham — the one who got plunged by my pal. He said his name, and one of the girls I was with said, "Oh I know him — he wouldn't do that, he's lovely."

Some 35 years after the Micky Droy testimonial, I had the good fortune to become good mates with a man who'd written a couple of football books. We met over something totally unrelated — dogs and clobber.

Strangely, we both knew who each other were. He'd been told to stay away from me — apparently, I was an arrogant prick who wouldn't sell him a dog. And I'd heard he'd written a paragraph about a mate of mine who'd passed in 2007 — who wasn't able to admit or deny the comment.

I mentioned on a hooligan Facebook page what Arsenal had done that night at the Micky Droy testimonial. Kingy's reply was short and sharp:

**"NEVER HAPPENED."

Off the back of that, we started chatting — me explaining that I'm not a liar, and him realising he'd been listening to a bunch of jealous pricks who'd told him I was an arrogant bastard who wouldn't sell him a dog. Turns out, he should've bought a puppy from me years ago — might've saved us both a lot of grief and a few Facebook rows.

I wasn't letting the Micky Droy night go. And as luck would have it, Kingy was chatting to a well-known Chelsea Head-hunter from Islington — another one who'd written a book. Kingy mentioned what I'd said, and the reply came back sharp as anything:

"They did."

That was enough for me.

We became great friends after that — proper mates. I still stay in touch with his partner Jan. There isn't a day that goes by I don't miss him.

He had a wicked sense of humour, a sharp tongue, and a heart the size of South/West London. He gave me stick, I gave it back, and somehow, we ended up laughing about dogs, clobber, and the night Arsenal ran riot at a Chelsea testimonial.

I've even made a few good pals at Chelsea and other clubs through Kingy — which just goes to show, even in a world built on rivalry, respect still counts.

God rest in eternal peace, my friend. You were one of the good ones — even if you were wrong about the Micky Droy night.

Chapter 18: Jasper Thompson

Jasper is the author of FUN, GAMES & HARD TIMES.

My Life as a football lad & Battle with FND.

First of all, I am happy Alan asked me to write a piece for him. I really appreciate it. Thanks, mate.

My name is Jasper Thompson and I was born in 1972. I was brought up in a small town called Heckmondwike which is about eight miles from Huddersfield, seven from Bradford and nine miles from Leeds. There was no doubt who I was going to support, my family and friends were all staunch Huddersfield Town fans. As a kid I remember the pitch battles at our old Leeds Road ground with Leeds, Manchester City, Sunderland, Newcastle, Chelsea, Millwall and Portsmouth. I was filled with fear/excitement but absolutely obsessed by it all. Over the years I have witnessed and been involved with various lads and different groups connected to Huddersfield Town. Like all mobs we won some, lost some and maybe had a few draws along the way. The best mobs I've come up against in no particular order were Bradford, Barnsley, Sheffield United, Sunderland, Bolton, Man City, Stoke and Birmingham. Been some top battles with them over the years. I'll go to the odd game but I don't like the culture anymore. It's a very different type of football I grew up with, I suppose success always brings in the tourists. I wish we could go back in time to the eighties and early nineties. Huddersfield were shit but the days out were awesome.

I first got to know Alan on social media. We would talk about our conditions and mental health etc. We have both been affected with the ability to walk properly. I really feel sorry for this guy. I know it's going to be a hard time for him and a long battle ahead. When we did meet, we instantly hit it off and had a great day out.

Alan is one of these guys, genuine and great company. Alan has moved over to Germany now, but even though we have our conditions we both ask each other if we are ok.

In 2010 I was diagnosed with Functional Neurological Disorder (FND). FND is the nervous system not working properly and a problem with the brain not receiving messages from the body. I was in and out of hospitals and in a wheelchair for four years. Symptoms are mainly functional limb weakness, functional walking problems, tiredness/spasms, speech/hearing loss, loss of memory and blackouts. I also fell into darkness and depression. I'm out of the wheelchair now and get about a bit with the aid of a walking stick. Of all the fights I've been involved in over the years, my battle with FND and mental health is far the toughest. My FND symptoms and mental health issues haven't gone away. I just want to live and manage my condition as best I can. Twenty-odd years ago asking for help was a sign of weakness. The sad thing is there's lot of sufferers in all walks of life. My message is this, it doesn't make you weak or inferior, you don't have to suffer in silence. Men have a high rate of suicide in this country and of course this as to change. You never know what someone is dealing with behind closed doors. No matter how happy someone looks, how loud their laugh is, or how big their smile is, there can always be a level of indescribable hurt. So be kind, even when others are not.

For my partner Janine. Life has been cruelled to me in many ways but no matter how hard it is and the pain I suffer, I have one amazing woman by my side to thank.

I've heard all the nonsense about Arsenal's mob being called the invisible firm act. In the eighties and early nineties, they were rated and one of the best dressed mobs around. Well-respected lads will vouch for that. I first came across the Arsenal mob after a match in London in the early-mid eighties. They were around a hundred handed and certainly looked the business. In 93 we had Arsenal in the League Cup. The first leg at ours we got stuffed 5-0 and at the return leg at Highbury we beat them 1-0. Arsenal's ground was a special place steeped in football history. Then in 2011 we had Arsenal away in the FA Cup. Don't get me wrong the Emirates is a fantastic stadium, but if it wasn't for the Town fans you would be able to hear a pin drop. Town played really well that day and rattled Arsenal but lost the game 2-1. After the match we nearly had it with Arsenal's mob outside their main pub the George but the police stopped it. I then came across Arsenal's mob one weekend away with the missus down London. I was impressed by Arsenal who were battling with Birmingham around King's Cross Station. They might not be as active as they were, but like most mobs when the big games come around, they will put on a show.

I think it's brilliant what Alan is doing with the book. I think he has completely nailed it. This book should be a must read not just for football fans but for us men who aren't good at expressing our thoughts and feelings with one another. I wish him the best of luck with it.

Chapter 19: Anderlecht's BCS

Our last battle with an English side in London was Arsenal back in 2014.

It was November and the first leg was in London.

Personally, I believe things in England are far from what they used to be back in the day but London is London and we rallied the troops for the trip across the channel.

We had a good 150 lads; at the time we were in good shape but nobody really knew what to expect from the Londoners.

The meeting point was the King's Cross St Pancras area where we had all booked our hotels.

We were split into around 10 hotels around the area and we kept our eyes open but all remained peaceful.

At the ground it was pretty much the same and there was nothing to write home about. All quiet on the hooligan front so far.

A well-known Cardiff top boy and a friend of mine was with us that day and he offered to set it up with Arsenal as he had a reliable contact there. 'Be my guest!' Was my eager reply.

I was curious, would Arsenal show up or was it just the usual blah-blah.

We returned to King 'Cross St Pancras and hit a few pubs but contrary to Brussels they closed relatively early and some of our lads wandered off.

It was already past midnight, and Arsenal were nowhere to be seen, though on the phone they kept saying they were coming.

Our numbers dwindled, many thought Arsenal would not be turning up any more and left, but I stayed there with a small group of 15-20 lads.

We had to be there in case Arsenal did eventually make a move. And they did.

Out of the blue a mob of them turned up and called it on. It was dark and to be honest at that stage we were not too attentive so it is difficult to accurately estimate their numbers but my educated guess is they were around 30, maybe 35. Credit to them, they came in hard and fast and took us a bit off guard.

What I liked less was that many of them were brandishing bottles.

Our frontliners were all among that 15-strong group and we had seen it all before so we just stood our ground.

A lad next to me got a bottle on his nut and started pissing claret,

Arsenal moved forward and we clashed. Some of our lads hit the tarmac, so did some of them but we held the line until more of our lads came out of their hotel lobbies to swell our numbers. In the end we were able to fight Arsenal off until the cops arrived and everybody fucked off sharply.

I am well aware that what follows is subject to interpretation, but I would leave it at a draw, but their lot was well up for it.

On a final note, I have a few observations. Firstly, had Arsenal turned up earlier as promised they would have had to face 150 lads instead of 20 and that would have meant a lot of trouble for them.

I assume they were in the know of what a firm we had; they must have had their scouts which is probably why they turned up later when our numbers had shrunk. Fair enough, it is all part of the game. And speaking of "game", Arsenal were as game as they come, though I don't think they needed all that glass.

(please forgive me for the pun). Anyway, their turf, their rules.

By and large it was a good ruck, so much is true. That said, the second leg in Brussels was a bit of a letdown.

We were expecting more but honestly nothing much happened.

We offered several locations where we could sort things out away from the watchful eye of police and CCTV.

Unfortunately, it turned out to be a long list of no-shows.

Arsenal was nowhere to be seen, I guess they had their reasons for not coming.

(To add to this section by Dave, there are always two sides to every story and we had a terrific mob in Brussels for the away game. We were plotted up about 15 minutes from the main square, we believed it to be called the Arab quarter, Anderlecht knew where we were because of their spotter who was constantly walking around outside, watching the gaff we were in and making calls. They never showed and it was time to leave the bar and at the square in an attempt to get at a mob of Anderlecht, Arsenal were sprayed with gas by the old bill. Arsenal was extremely disappointed that Anderlecht never showed up)

Summing up, I have mixed feelings about Arsenal. On one hand they did better than Spurs or Chelsea when we had them but on the other, we were hoping for more.

On a personal level I would like to add that back in 2006 I had travelled with a couple of mates to London for a football weekend.

On Saturday April 22 Arsenal had Spurs home in what was going to be the last North London derby at Highbury, a historical moment I wanted to enjoy with some BCS mates. We hit a pub and got talking with some blokes who turned out to be in the know. On the funny side some of them spoke French as they had Congolese origins.

They were seasoned Arsenal lads, I guess from Denton's crew and we had a nice chat and bevvied.

Their firm made a good impression on me to be honest and I guess so did we, though we were just a handful.

Dave BCS Anderlecht.

Chapter 20: More Than Just a Tear Up

The stories I've written about include no names — just events I was at, moments I lived, and things I can be called out for. But this book has a purpose. As I said in the foreword, it's not a book about hooliganism. It's about survival. It's about identity. It's about how a tough upbringing, a fractured world, and a need to belong shaped who I became.

No matter what your thoughts are on fighting, I've written it like this for a reason. Because behind every punch thrown was a story. Behind every chase, every scar, every roar from the terraces — there was a kid trying to find his place.

I could carry on writing for what feels like forever.

I could talk about jumping on a coach in 1983 outside the Champion boozer in Upper Street to go down to Portsmouth. They'd always been shit — lower divisions, no real history with us. But this was a pre-season friendly, and we'd heard Spurs or West Ham had been down there and come off worse. The real reason? Charlie Nicholas. The club had fought hard to sign him from Celtic, and we all had to see him.

Pompey didn't rate Arsenal — like many others at the time. But they had the shock of their lives when we broke out of police escorts and chased them through side streets. They knew who we were after that. Turnstiles got done in the mayhem, and a few of ours earned a few quid that day.

Funniest part? Queuing up in a sleepy village near Leatherhead — proper queuing, like good citizens — for fizzy drinks, crisps, and chocolate. Then one lad says, "Fuck this," and walks out with his arms full. Well, that place got emptied like a swarm of locusts had hit it.

Two cars of local bobbies turn up to a couple of coaches full of louts. They start taking names. One lad puts on a thin Scouse accent and gives a Birmingham address. The copper says, “I love your accent — unmistakable.” Cue more laughter and piss-taking.

We all got back on the coach. A copper — looked about 12 — gets on and says, “The petrol station manager won’t press charges if you just give back what you took.” He says he’ll be back in a couple of minutes.

I expected everything to be down the front of the coach. But while he was chatting bollocks to the other coach, everyone on ours was stuffing themselves with chocolate and crisps, chucking the empty wrappers down the front.

We all sat there like innocent schoolkids. On pops kindergarten cop to a mountain of wrappers and 52 lads trying not to laugh — some still chewing, others looking green.

He looked up, smiled, and said: **“FUCK OFF. JUST GO.”**

I could talk about failed attempts by Spurs and West Ham to infiltrate the North Bank — and getting caned each time. Or going to Spurs in the early ’80s and going at the Bull pub. They didn’t come out until we’d passed — then tried to come out behind us. We turned and had a war. We claimed the bragging rights that day.

Or the much-documented Battle of Highbury when Millwall came to us. The Islington Gazette made it sound like they tore through the borough like a marauding Viking army. But I could tell it from our side — where we ran them up and down Blackstock Road. Or the incident in Highbury Fields, where the famous Bushwackers made a tactical retreat into Highbury & Islington tube station.

I was told personally by one of the well-respected Millwall men — of Panorama fame — that when we went at them and a black geezer clumped SM out of Eltham, they thought he was dead the way he went over and cracked his head. He said, "We never thought Arsenal were that good."

I could write about going to West Ham and taking it to them in their own ground. Or watching them run along the train tracks to get away from us.

Or Galatasaray in Copenhagen — well documented and filmed. The tension in the air was unreal. The Turks had killed two Leeds fans two weeks before in the semi-final. Scumbags even hit a bond with a chair while he was giving CPR to one of the stabbing victims.

Loads of my pals went out the day before. I went early on match day. Up at 4am to get to Gatwick for the first flight.

Made a coffee, stuck the news on — and there they were. Clips of my mates fighting outside a restaurant. Bleeding. Severely outnumbered.

One of them was so bloody I didn't even recognise him — and I'd known him since I was 10.

I called one of the lads when we landed. He said, "Stay away from the square."

We got off the bus and within seconds, I had the most laughable thing imaginable happen to me. An old grey-haired Turk grabbed my jacket and started hitting me with his shoe. Brown shiny suit, fag hanging out of his mouth — whacking me with his shoe like I was a naughty grandchild. It must've looked hilarious.

We met in a big Irish boozer near the square. From memory, the bouncers asked us to drink upstairs — the Turks were looking like they'd do all the windows.

We had a quiet drink upstairs while any Arsenal shirt outside was a target. Then the shout went up — and we came out swinging.

Straight across the road into them. I was beside one of the Herd's main men — still respected to this day. He took one on the nose and was bleeding. I got hit with a chair that broke my left thumb. I just squeezed it while typing this — it's never been right in 25 years.

I didn't eat a kebab for seven years after that.

It was Arsenal who did the damage to the Turks that day — even though four of ours were stabbed. No other English alliance there. No one else turned up for revenge. Just us.

For Chris and Kevin — the Leeds lads who never made it home. Rest in peace.

There's so much more I could write about that trip — and about the great adventure in Paris against PSG.

A city that big with one football club. No one took it to PSG — especially not in 1994. They were terrorising everyone. They'd already had the mighty Chelsea Head-hunters over.

But we didn't give two fucks. We were Arsenal.

I was living in Kent by then. Me and my pal jumped on an Archway coach organised by a superstar running a boozer in Finchley.

We took the short journey to grand Paris. Stopped at some lights. An English copper got on and gave us advice:

"When you turn the next corner, you'll be kept in the car park until you're taken to the ground. It's for your own safety."

TISSSSSHHHHHH. All the emergency handles were pulled. The coach emptied. The one behind did the same.

We were off.

We battled with PSG for what felt like hours. After the game, there weren't many of us without cuts and bruises.

I could tell some great stories about the extent that we went too to be known as the best dressed firm in England and taxing of bods out shopping or being taxed outside Knick Knacks or Selfridges, Cobras Sports, west London, venturing to the High Road in N17 to Stag Sports and hoping not to be recognised, trying to do pay weekly deals with George and Athos who owned Cult on Camden Road, the deal was. Can I please pay weekly for my next Sergio Tacchini tracked suit.

If a northern mob came to us dressed how we dressed, we made sure that next time we were well in front of the, switching to Jaeger, Valentine, Cerruti etc.

I could go on. I could write another hundred pages. The buzz, the violence, the madness — it's endless. But that's not what this book is really about.

It's about what shaped me. What shaped us. The chaos, the brotherhood, the fear, the pride. The fight to belong. The fight to survive.

This isn't a book about hooliganism. It's a book about life — and what it takes to come through it swinging.

I've lived through more than just fights and football. Behind the buzz, the blood, and the brotherhood was something darker — a world where loyalty was tested, trust was currency, and silence was survival. During those years, some of the hooligans branched out — took the natural step into the grimy world of crime. I won't go into too much detail. I'm not here to be judged. But as the late 80s and early 1990s rolled in, I wasn't seen at football as much.

I was into other things. I'm not Paul Sykes — I haven't swum the Straits of Doha in white pumps — but I've lived. I've written about my experiences. I've sat at the tables of Mafia men in New Jersey, and equally at the table of a Mafia family in Sicily — the kind where if you are at the dinner table and say you're full, the lady of the house keeps feeding you, and her husband simply says, “Eat.” So, I ate.

I was used by a northern mob as a debt collector to get what was owed to them by others in a different City, not because the northerners were scared of cockneys, they used me purely because it was a different entity thrown into the ring.

Their logic was that if a cockney gets involved, the mob owing the debt will not know how well connected you are, who you are and how big the damage can become.

I would calmly and nonchalantly say things like, I don’t need this petty squabbling, it’s way too much grief, I just want wants owed and I can stay in the background, and everyone is happy.

I could go into what the consequences would be if you carry on playing these games, but I would imagine that you are experienced enough to not have me waste my time with threats.

It usually worked.

I had to carry out this task based on the fact that one of my bods was robbed and I was paying off a debt.

It didn’t on one occasion, but that’s for another time.

There is one quick story, when I managed to get away for this life, I moved to the Kent coast and got a plot to breed my Dogue de Bordeaux’s, Cane Corso and American Bulldogs.

The next-door neighbour sees this big old lump, the Harley Davidson parked on the drive, the first thing that I did was get some builders to build to brick peers and fit electric 6ft metal gates and I also never went to work much (in her eyes) but I had my own business and while my labour was on site, I was winning the work and managing it.

I explained that we moved down there to bring up a family in a nicer environment and I had the business and this seemed to appease the nosey outspoken old trout until the phone call.

I am down at the kennels and Luc shouts out "DAD, DAD its Paul on the phone, come up now, he doesn't have long."

My reply was simple, tell him that I will ring him back, my brother is called Paul and due to personal reasons needed me.

Lucs reply: at full voice NO ITS PAUL RINGING FROM PRISON SO HURRY UP.

The nosey neighbour was in her garden and heard it all.

It's been a life. Complicated. Scary. But fun.

A life of dangerous liaisons with dangerous people. Dodgy deals and deceptions.

"I came up in a time and place that shaped me in ways no outsider could ever truly grasp. The chaos of the terraces, the violence in the schools, the rush of living on the edge—it was a world that made sense only to those who were there. I did what I did for reasons that belong to me alone, and trying to explain them to anyone else would be pointless. I carry no regrets, because regret would mean denying the truth of who I was. I meant no harm, and I never set out to be anything more than part of the movement around me. In the end, I followed the HERD."

Alan Bates

PART TWO

Chapter 21: Bow Legged

I tell you what, I absolutely hate squeaky floors and when I say I hate squeaky floors, it's almost like someone eating loudly and you're sitting there looking at them and you want to kill them. That's how much I hate squeaky floors. So, I bought this gaff right out in the middle of nowhere. You know, I'd been breeding the dogs, needed that bit more space. So, after all the years of working to get the dog to Bordeaux recognized in England, in the UK, you know, I needed to be out in the middle of nowhere. So got the dog set up, got all the kennels, built all the concrete and done got the run set up. So, if one dog didn't like another dog, even his little group could be on one side, the other group can be on the other. So, the dogs were over the moon. But me, all I could hear every time I was watching the telly was a squeaking upstairs. Or if you got up in the middle of the night for a tinkle, straight away all you could hear was the noise and you felt like from where I was, you could hear it in Paris.

Anyway, I get this idea. I'll tell you what I'm going to do. I'm going to rip all them epoxy carpets up, I'm going to go down B and Q, I'm going to get all the gear, there aren't going to be no more squeaky floors. Not for me, no more squeaky floors. So, get all the gear, all the carpets are up, pull all the floors up. Standing on these joists, absolutely lovely, having a look around, what I got to do. I'm going to put a bit of extra bit there, I'm going to put an extra bit there, going to make it as solid as a rock less floor. So just as I turn, there's a little nail in the floor. Bang. One foot goes straight through the ceiling, downwards. My right foot, instead of bending how you'd expect your right, your right knee to bend, it bent sideways, so pulled all the cartilage off my knee. As I've gone over, I've hit me head on the newel post, smashed me head to bits. Now I'm lying there unconscious, leg dangling through above the cooker.

It was a right sight. Smashed a bit, absolutely smashed. So later that day, me pal comes around, he's doing some flaws, my pal Grant, and he just could not stop laughing. I had one of them lumps, you know, like on Tom and Jerry, when Jerry gets it on the head and the lump comes up and it goes through his hair and it Sticks up. I had a lump like that on my head and he could not stop laughing at me. So next day, knees a bit sore. Day after that I could hardly walk, swelling come up it was unbearable.

Well, that was the start of my trauma. That has got me now, twenty odd years later to where I am.

That poxy knee, I go in, I have certain things done to it. I have cortisone injections; I have fluid drained off.

This is over a twenty-year period, but even when I went in and see the doctor on that very first day that I pulled it apart and it was all smashed up and he'd done a little bit of surgery on it, he said, in about twenty years, when you're in your mid-fifties, you're going to need a new knee.

So I went, all right then, fair enough, but it's going to be all right for now. He said, well, you're going to have moments. It's going to get worse and worse over the years, but you're all right, you can go for now. So off I pop, keep having me injections. Over the years, everything's fine, I get to my mid-fifties, right? The Doctor timed it perfectly.

Although I was always a fat fucker. I've done all the training, all the kickboxing and everything else, but I was always relatively healthy. As soon as that knee popped on that, when I had that fall, it all becomes shit. I lasted as long as I could without knee pain. I got maybe mid-forties, had to go in, have different injections done, had to have cortisone put in my knee again.

Then I had a surgery which was a clean out, bits of fragmented bone in the left knee. So, get all booked in, go and have it done. Lovely jubbly, all as good as gold.

About four weeks after the surgery, I contacted the surgeon and said that I want to pop over to the wife's parents in Spain. Is it all right to fly now? Yeah, yeah, yeah, of course you can, of course you can. Go on, get on the flight, enjoy yourself, try and relax. So, I get out there, I'm all strapped up, my knees still strapped up.

I'm being very, very, very cautious, so we have a nice little break, come back and I've got this horrible, horrible pain in my left calf.

I go in to see this physiotherapist called Faye in Chelmsford. She's massaging the leg, doing deep tissue massage.

Then I go back another day and she's now sticking big needles into the calf to try and break up the muscle because the muscles got really tight, in her opinion.

She was probably sticking the big needles in me because she was a season ticket holder at Spurs.

So, I'm in absolute agony. but you don't think nothing of it.

The reason you don't think nothing of it is because you're in a position where you've had surgery, right? You're sitting around doing not a lot and it's the same leg that you've had the surgery on and then you've got a qualified physiotherapist with a degree tell you that it's because your calf muscles gone really tight and it's almost in a situation where it's in a cramp feeling all the time.

One Friday night I'm lying there and I say, I've got go to bed, my leg's killing me.

So, all night I'm struggling and the pain is intense, real, real intense pain.

I'm awake four o' clock in the morning, go downstairs.

When the missus gets up, I say to her, can we pop into town, get a Costa or something? I've got to get out the house, because This is sending me mad. The highlight of my days, when you come home from work and I'm just struggling, really, really struggling. I've got to get out the house. She says, are you all, right? Yeah, of course. I'm just my legs playing me up a bit. We get in the car, go to Costa, start drinking my coffee and I start coughing and then its proper violent coughing and I'm now coughing in a way that you can't draw a breath.

People in the Costas are looking at me, Bianca's panicking and I'm coughing and believe me, when I say I'm coughing, I am coughing. It's a dry, nasty, horrible cough and I've got this pain in my chest.

Everyone assumes at this stage I'm having a heart attack. So having this really, really, really nasty feeling, can't get me breath and I am looking Bee with that goodbye look in my eyes.

This goes on for a good few minutes and then it passes and you think, we got to get home, we've really got to get home. So, we get in the car, Bianca gets me home and calls the emergency doctor's line on a Saturday, go in and see him and he basically gives me the once over and says, basically, don't know what it is, it was just a coughing attack and go home, try and get some rest.

So, we go home and do as I am told and that night, we're sitting in the house and I feel bad, I feel so bad, my head's gone, I am bright red, my eyes are rolling in my head and it comes to the stage where, no, this is serious now, we better call an ambulance.

Bianca calls an ambulance, the paramedics come in, they take my blood pressure and it's literally through the roof.

They check me for a stroke as that is what my symptoms were showing and as I hadn't stroked, they were expecting one.

They get me in the back of the ambulance and boom, I'm blue lighted into Chelmsford.

So, it turns out that that coughing fit was a massive blood clot that broke up, thankfully, thank the lords above, that broke up, passed through my heart and wedged in each of the two lungs in the tubes going into the two lungs. Now, if it had stayed the same size and moved, it would have killed me instantly.

That's exactly what happened to my mum, when we come back from holiday, she complained about feeling rough the way I was complaining about feeling rough while we were on holiday. She comes back and on Friday and on the Sunday night she was ironing my dad's clothes and took a big cough, took a deep breath and she was dead before she hit the floor.

Now I would have been in the Same position, but luckily this clot broke and it passed through all the tubes, passed through the heart and boom, I survived it.

So, we go through months and months of warfarin. Not Wolverine, the film Wolverine. Backwards and forwards to hospitals and then the doctors come up with this idea.

We're going to find out if it's hereditary because of your mom's history and your granddad's history, and once we find out whether it's hereditary or not, then we can make a decision on what we're going to do for treating you for the future.

I didn't stop the warfarin straight away because we were going to Egypt over the new year.

Anyway, six weeks after all this, we go through into January, and then I get the call, can you come in and see the doctor at Orsett Hospital? Go in there, got good news, sir. This is not hereditary. It's just one of them things that happened through the course of the surgery and there's no need for any more medication, so all's good. Be on your way and live your life, so, I was on my way and started living my life.

Come the April that year, March, April, I left Canary Wharf and took on a new job at a company called McLarens. I started there on the Monday, and by the Friday, I couldn't get up the stairs in the office, I managed to get to the top but stood outside the office until I managed to get my breath back until I was feeling alright to go in the office, went in the office, bluffed it, didn't go out to lunch because I knew that I wouldn't be able to get back up the stairs.

So, I stayed in the office all day, called the wife and said, look, something is not right. Can you get me an emergency appointment? I really need to get in and see a doctor. I managed to get my way back, see the doctor, she does my saturations for my blood, writes me a letter and says to me, can you get to Basildon Hospital immediately? Because they say it's not right and I'm just worrying whether there's another pulmonary embolism in your lungs.

So, I said, yeah, yeah, no worries, no worries. But me being me, we'd already booked to go to Miller and Carter, the one on the, on the boat, lakeside. So, I said to my misses you know, the doctors said, get to the hospital straight away, but it's going to be rammed. It's six o'clock on a Friday night. It's going to be rammed. Let's get up about four in the morning, then that way everyone who's been in a bar fight or hurt themselves on Friday night has been dealt with at the hospital. We're going there to be dead quiet. So, she just couldn't believe what she was hearing. I said, plus, I'm due a pint of Peroni. I've had a hard week. First week at the new company and not felt so good, so. So, let's go and have a nice bit of dinner. So, against her wishes, we went down, we had our dinner, went to bed that night, got up about four o', clock and made our way to the hospital, probably in the hospital about five o', clock, got seen to after a couple of hours and the doctor calls me in, says, come and have a look at this, Mr Bates.

He shows me the screen and there is an absolutely massive clot right next to my heart and the wording was, if that moves, you're gone. So, what do you mean, if that moves, you're gone. He said, if that moves, you're no longer with us. So, I was instantly admitted into the ICU and that was the start of my health issues going forward, but believe me, those couple of Peronis and a bit of medium rare Joe Blake were handsome.

As the years pass, it apparent that I need a new knee.

So, I go to the hospital. And the doctor confirms that I need a new knee.

We're going to do it January second, all planned.

Honestly, never realized what this was going to be like. So go in and the doctor does the knee and then I go through the next few months of hell. So, if any of your lot, I know a few of you reading this have had your knees done, well, hopefully a few of you will read it, who have had your knees done, don't it fucking hurt.

They butcher ya. And when you see the tools, it is unbelievable.

Funny thing is that the doctor was a season ticket holder at Watford and always had me in stitches about football.

At this time, I severely hated Wenger and he adored him, anyone who weren't an Arsenal fan who supported a smaller team was in ore of Arsene Wenger, but I couldn't even listen to him be interviewed anymore.

We had a nice Christmas in Germany and prepared for the day of surgery on the 2nd of January and it's not like the NHS, having Bupa through work, unless the surgeon is sick or falls off of his bike on the way to work, we are having it done.

The anaesthetist was quite funny and he showed me bits of bone afterwards and he, you know, he showed me all different things and he calls his role in the surgery, the gin and tonic lounge, because they don't actually put you out. What they do when they've got the nasty bits, when there's drills, hammers and chisels, they're smashing you about, they turn it up a bit so you go sleep. Then they turn it down a bit so your kind of with it and not if that makes sense.

Knee gets done, I'm out, sorted, rocking and rolling. So as time goes by, the left one's playing up. We always knew the left one was playing up because I'll tell you what, when I was standing, standing still, I looked like Malcolm McDonald or an old Jacky Chan.

If someone let a pig go in a passage, it run straight through my legs when my ankle's touching. That's how bad my knees were.

So, now I've got one straight one which is handsome.

The doctors done a really good job on it and I've got this other one that's all pissed and bent, but what was happening was over a period of time, I would be walking along and I felt like me, my hips were playing up and every now and again I was always leaning on things or stopping for a rest when I went out on site.

I'd go upstairs and stop but I put that down to my weight. I thought because I'm a big lump, you know, it's my, my legs can't handle the weight, my back, my hips can't handle the weight, something couldn't handle the weight.

I got to the stage where I didn't know what it was but I started shitting myself literally, not like cowardly shitting myself, but the full monty.

Things would happen and I just couldn't hold my poo.

I just thought that was a food thing, so instead of going back to the doctor that done my right knee because I thought it was my hips and it was happening at my lower back.

I went in and see this professor, a nice funny Singaporean Chinese mam who had me in stitches all the time as he was a character and his son was an avid Arsenal fan.

It seems that everything comes down to football with me.

So, we talked about all different things. Good as gold going and see him and so I explained to him what was going on, thought my hips were playing up and I come and see him because he was a professor that dealt with hips and knees.

That's why I didn't go back to the other doctor because he'd just did knees.

So, I thought this doctor was going to play about with my hips and knees and all that good stuff.

So gone in and see this him and he lays me on my back, lifts my leg up, pulls my leg round, pulls the other one round, puts his weight on both knees so they go flat.

So, I lean back, pulls me around and he says, I tell you what, you've got hips like a fifty-five-year-old ballerina.

So, I thought handsome, nothing wrong with my hips.

He said there is nothing wrong with your lower back, but I will tell you what we do, we'll we get some scans done anyway.

The news was that my left knee is in a bad way.

He said that you always knew you needed your left knee done because it was bad when you got your right knee done.

So, let's get your knee done and we worry about your back later because I can't see anything wrong with your hips.

Your hips are fine. They're moving around, they're not grinding, there's no arthritis in there at all, so we an appointment, we go in to get my knee done in October.

I am sitting there and the anaesthetist comes in and they attempt the epidural.

So, like I said before, they don't actually knock you out under a general anaesthetic.

So, I am sitting on the table and geezer goes in with a needle.

I nearly hit the roof. I've never felt pain like it. So, he quickly pulled the needle out. He said, oh, oh, I've caught a nerve. To fucking right he caught a nerve. So, I'm sitting there and he said, are you all, right? So, I said, well, not really.

I've never felt anything like that in my life. So, he calls a nurse in, a male nurse sees I'm sitting there, so I'm all lent forward, curled over a bit, and I've got this nurse holding both my shoulders in a way that I won't fall off the table if I passed out.

So, it goes in again, honestly, immediate sweat. Never felt anything like this. So, they've had two attempts now to get in.

So, they've hit my nerve in, in my spine twice.

He goes in, talks to the professor.

The professor comes out and sees me, says, look, we can't go down the route that we're going to.

I said, well, you're still doing the operation. He said, yeah, but with your permission, we do a general anaesthetic. I said, I don't care what you do.

We're ready for it now. Let's go and do it. So, I go and do the surgery, wake up.

Normal pain that you have with having your knee done. From what I've been told, it's the most painful recovery of any surgery that they do in hospitals. They reckon it's up there with the best of them.

So you go through your hell, you're bending, you're stretching, you're doing your physio, you're doing everything you're meant to do.

You're doing ice packs; you're doing warm packs.

I'm doing everything that I learned from the first knee that I had done...

I rented a machine that that you strapped your leg into that bent your leg back and it done it every so many seconds or every so many minutes. So, I did everything that you were meant to do to get back to Normal as best you can with two metal knees.

Over a period of time, I'm getting there, as previously mentioned, the surgery was in October.

Now we are coming up to Christmas, I'm really bad and also sad. Never been sad like this before.

Obviously, all blokes get sad, but not like it's taking over your life.

I'm thinking that I've got two new knees, I'm moving around, all that pain's gone. I'm an inch taller again, so that's good, Where the bow legs have gone straight.

The problem is that I'm not getting better.

My knees got better or were Getting better, after six, eight weeks of having your knee done, you're moving around, a lot of the pain starts to go.

It takes a few months, but a lot of the pain starts to go and you should be in a good position, but I'm not.

So, what we do is our annual Christmas stay in Germany as my father in law's birthday is on Christmas day.

We never miss a Christmas in Germany, so we drive over and I'm in a proper bad way.

It's my hips again.

I've been told by that professor there's nothing wrong with me hips and it weren't my back because my back wasn't hurting.

We're in Germany and I'm living off of painkillers, I'm taking whatever I can, within reason, so you don't overdo it.

Nothing's happening. I'm sad, I can't get up and I can't hold my poo and I'm dribbling a lot when I wee and I'm thinking there's got to be something not right there.

We managed to get an appointment with a physiotherapist, just after Christmas day. But let's go back a step. On Christmas morning I could not get out of bed.

Now it's my father in law's birthday but ultimately, it's Christmas and at that time I had a three-year-old Son and not being able to get out of bed was heartbreaking, not just for me and Bee, but for Henry.

All the family forgave me, not that there was anything to forgive.

I was, I was quite ill. I could not get out of bed. I laid on the bed in darkness all day long listening to several families like brother-in-law and cousins and all that stuff.

Visitors came in all day,

I Laid in total darkness and a depression had come over me. I couldn't really get up.

I had two new knees. Which in itself means that I'd gone through a couple of years of hell with having the knees done and I couldn't get up.

I had no strength; there was nothing there. So luckily enough, I had the, the professor on WhatsApp. So, I banged him a text and I told him what was going on and he said, look, it's not your knees and it weren't your rips.

He said, when you come back, I'll book you an appointment. Now, when you're back in England, go and get an MRI done. So, this physiotherapist in Germany, he starts to work on me, bends me knee, right knee, and he says, oh, that one's doing really well. Bends the left knee. Bear in mind, I'm only two months in, so I can't, can't go mad with a left knee.

He bends my left knee, tests all around both legs and he says to my missus, there's nothing wrong with his legs because with what I've just done to him, if there was something wrong with his legs, he would have hit the roof by now.

So, there's nothing wrong with his knees.

He goes up me back and he's crunching away and he's having a little feel around and he touched me around chest level, nipple level on your back and it Took my breath away immediately.

He then he did it again and I was asked he not to do it again.

It was just odd, the oddest feeling. Similar to when the, the anaesthetist stuck the needle in my nerve.

He said that you really need to get this checked out when you get back to England, because I don't know what that is, but there's something there and I've never experienced anything like that before, touching someone there and them having that reaction.

When we got back, we got an emergency MRI done and my professor, the knee professor, looks at the, the MRI and he says, look, I'm not a back specialist nut I know a great Doctor who is and I will refer you.

A neurosurgeon that I was referred to is very well thought of and very up to date with all modern technologies and everything in his field of speciality.

Let's let him have a look at it.

So, one Saturday morning comes round and he says to me, I go in and see him. Sit down, Mr Bates, got some news for you.

I thought, oh, this don't sound good and he says, you've got spinal dural arteriovenous fistulas in your back. So, I said OK and then he said, well, we're very lucky to have found it. You're very lucky to have come to me because he was obviously clearly an arrogant man.

He loved himself a little bit as neurosurgeons do, they feel like they're godlike figures.

So, you're very lucky you come to me because most neurosurgeons wouldn't have found this. And then he showed me the MRI and he showed me the little dots, and he talked me through what fistulas are, they're malformations of blood vessels.

I asked what's the outcome of this? He said, well, if that ruptures, you'll be paralyzed from your chest down.

What?

Then obviously, the room went silent. And I sat there and my eyes filled up with water, and he's looking at me and I said, well, what's the likelihood of that happening?

He said, well, it's very likely it could happen, but what I need to do, I need a better-quality MRI.

I need you to go to a radiologist and get this looked at properly and then we will see what we can do.

We will get you in for surgery, but the surgery will be to see if we can do an embolization, which Is gluing a certain place to get the blood flows running properly.

So, I said, okay, when are we going to get this done? So, he said, well, I'm going to get you down for an emergency MRI. So maybe two, three days later, we were in for. I was in for an emergency MRI.

I will tell you what, this was a long one. A proper, proper long one. So, laying there, listening to the boom, bang, shakalak rattling for what seemed like hours.

I think it was about hour and a half, ninety minute one. laying there thinking, this is strange I can't feel my legs, what's going on here?

The MRI finishes. It rolls me out. I'm laying now and the staff said you can get up now.

So, they sat me up and I said, I can't. I can't feel anything from my chest down. And they said, all right, just, you just sit there for a little while.

You'll be all right in a minute. Just get the blood flowing around a bit. So, they sat me up, spun me around, so my legs were hanging over the side the side of the contraption.

Nope, couldn't feel my legs, couldn't feel anything. So, they get a doctor, doctor comes in, tapping my legs, feeling my toes, nothing.

So now there's a bit of a panic. I'm in a private hospital in Brentwood, where the only way is Essex is filmed, and they had to call an ambulance.

The ambulance comes, gets me all sorted.

I am strapped up in the back of the ambulance, we're going off to a neurological ward in London, a specialist ward that deals with neurology and they're going to sort me out.

So, this is how lucky I am, lucky, Al.

We're in the ambulance, sitting in bit of traffic on the A12 on the Romford Road.

Bang. A motorbike goes over in front of us.

So, they say to me, do you mind if we stop and just deal with this motorbike? So, the police come, and a copper gets in the back of the ambulance and says are You all right there, mate? yeah, yeah, of course I am. So, they, they deal with the emergency.

The geezer who came off the bike gets sorted out while another ambulance comes and then we're off.

So, we go set off for the big boy's ward.

When we get there, it's shocking, security is walking around everywhere in stab vests and we wait in a corridor for a couple of hours to see triage and a nurse come over and says, we already know about you, you should have been taken to the ward ages ago.

I arrives on the ward an immediately realise that I am in a different world, the man in the bed opposite has got an air pipe in his throat.

He is staring at the ceiling. He's clearly in some sort of coma,

His heads switched off, and he's just breathing through this thing and his family come and they talk to him and they leave, and there's a geezer in the bed beside him in a very similar position. So, I'm now in the big time Charlie ward, the neurological world where people have had brain surgery, they've had their skull taken off, put back on again because they've had tumours taken out their brains and blah, blah, blah. There's a young fellow the other side of my curtain, I can hear him talking to his girlfriend and he says, look, babe, I'm in the neurological ward at Romford.

So, she must have said, what do you mean you're in a neurological ward? And it turns out he was. He got out of his van in the morning, he got to work and he passed out, right? So, the ambulance was called, they've took him into hospital, bang, he's got some sort of been down for scans.

He's got a tumour in his head, so they're going to be dealing with him. So, he's crying the other side of me, while talking to his bird, and I'm just on this bed and now I'm feeling like a proper fraud.

I've got this geezer with a tumour in his head and there's me just got a bit of an issue where someone's stuck a pin in me back and caught a nerve that caused a bit of problem.

Well, that is what thought and it turned out not to be that someone caught a nerve with a needle in my back and caught. It was nothing to do with that, but that's what my brain was still telling me but it was this spinal dural arteriovenous fistula.

They are part of what they call one of the rarest diseases in the world. A rare disease in any country has to be above two hundred thousand and then it is classed literally as a rare disease. In that range, two hundred thousand is a rare disease. Well, I live in Germany and we do it on the German stats. In Germany, you get anything up to four people per one point one million get this disease.

Forty percent of the people that get this disease are dead, and found at postmortem stage. Now we're now down to sixty percent. So, sixty percent of the four people at one point one million, so we're looking at three hundred and odd people get this disease out of 85 million.

So, it's a very, very, very rare disease.

I'm sitting there and it's really not dawned on me, what's actually wrong with me.

I can hear these machines, these pumping, getting the bloke opposite to breathe.

Later that night a young doctor who works in the Neurological team comes around, does all my stats, the standard stuff like blood pressure, all the different things, saturations etc. and he's talking away to me and I was wearing a really nice watch, a Panerai and this geezer was into Panerai's and watches in general.

We started chatting about watches and all that gear and he opened up and I said to him, this is a bit embarrassing, sitting here with all these people. He said, why is it embarrassing? I said, there's not a lot wrong with me compared to them. and he, turned around and made it very clear to me that there was a hell of a lot wrong with me.

Look at your surroundings, you are not in this ward because of lack of beds elsewhere, it is because you are very sick.

The next morning comes after a long night of feeling uncomfortable and feeling like I would piss myself amongst other things.

I had a little bit of feeling coming back, but not enough to walk.

Next morning they took me down to surgery.

The surgery was for the radiologist to see if they could go in and embolise the fistulas.

What the idea is they get the whole team together, the anaesthetist, the radiologist, etcetera and the whole team has to be certain that they can reach the fistulas, that they can embolize and do exactly what they believe needs doing, and that they will be able to do it safely in order solve the problem and I walk away. With the belief that I should be all right over a period of a few weeks. So, we go down, sign all the paperwork.

They said, you know that you could have a stroke, you could have this, you could die.

I signed the paperwork and then I went through something that I had never experienced before, when I've gone down for surgery before. You don't actually go in the operating theatre when you are awake.

You're normally sound asleep by the time you're near any surgeons or anything else.

They wheel me into this room. I've still got my underpants on, I've got one of their gowns on, they never told me to take me underpants off or nothing.

I really am confused and embarrassed, I don't really know what's going on and I am not really with it.

They say, could you get up and lay on that table? So, I said, my legs are not working properly. Oh, yeah, yeah, yeah. So, they lift me onto this table, this table has got a ruler that's designed into it, like a big, long measuring line.

Then they say, could you move up a bit? Now, bear in mind, my legs aren't working properly, I am twenty-three stone, then its, a bit more, So, you drag yourself up a bit. A little bit more. Little bit to the left, little bit to the right.

So now I've built up a sweat and I'm. I'm struggling, I feel uncomfortable. So, I'm lying there and one of the nurses, or the assistant theatre technician, says, you've still got your pants on.

Can you take them off?

I went, no, I can't. Can't you take them off?

You've just seen all that I've gone through to get to this.

So, there's. I'm now getting a bit worked up and I'm never rude to people.

I swear by trying to be nice to people and being a good person, anyway, so I'm lying there, I'm now got the indignity, if that's the word, of someone taking my underpants off.

I'm not the most blessed man in the world, I’ve got what looks like a tortoise head in a roll neck. So, it's very, very embarrassing, and it was all because when they do the radiology, they've got this machine that actually is almost seeing through you down to a measurement.

They have to know exactly where fistulas are for when they're doing their bit and they record stuff where the measurements are for next time.

So that's, that's all good. So, we're all chatting and we're all having a bit of a laugh.

The anaesthetist does his job. Very nice person.

A young Filipino nurse was there assisting the anaesthetist. She's chatting to me, what do you do for a living? Blah, blah, blah.

By the time you've actually answered what you do for a living, you're waking up in recovery and everything's fine.

No sickness, no sore throat from the whatever they put down your throat, everything's fine. They take me up to the ward, I'm back in bed and quite relaxed, everything's fine.

The doctor comes in and sees me and he says, we've had a meeting and we believe that we can reach the fistula. It's an awkward one and extremely complicated but we believe that we can reach it.

What he said to me was, if we can't reach it and we can't close it, we will have to open you up on Friday, we will have to do a full-scale operation, which means we cut your bone in half.

We get to your spine and They take it out section by section. They go in, they repair the fistula and they put the bone back on, put some screws and cement in and the fistula is fixed.

Then he says, if we can't get everything right tomorrow, we do that on Friday. So I went, okay, so we're fingers crossed that we're not going to do the open surgery, we do the embolization and it works.

The next day comes after a really rough night, it felt like they dropped me or when they dragged me across from the operating table, back onto the bed, that my elbow caught my ribs.

I just could not get comfortable; I was in incredible pain all night.

A lovely Jamaican nurse who comes in for the night shift was giving me painkillers, she was helping me get settled, making me some tea and all that stuff and then I said oh, I'm not meant to have tea. I'm having surgery in the morning; we had a bit of a laugh about that and the next morning comes after a hellish night.

I'm tired, I'm upset, I'm scared. I haven't seen my wife. It's hard, when you've got this rare disease.

They're trying something. If this don't work, it's a major operation. We're cutting your back bone in half and taking a section out,

So, yes, I'm scared.

During the journey down on the bed, I'm laughing and joking, doing what Alan does, having a bit of banter with them, bit of fun, they're all enjoying it, they roll me in. Can you get on the table? and now I know what I've got to do.

So, they get me on the table, got my paper underpants on, so they're just going to rip them off in a little while. So that's all, all sorted. We're all covered, pull myself about now.

That's not right. Could you go down a bit? So, you go back down, then its sideways.

It takes a bit of time to get where you need to be.

What's happened is today is that we haven't got the same anaesthetist.

We've got a locum or an agency man or whatever their called, but this man has the bedside manner of a concentration camp commandant.

This man is horrible and he stank of body odour.

He is tapping my left hand to put a needle in for his line and I said to him, look, mate, they tried this yesterday it doesn't really work, the left hand. I don't know why you're not going to get the flow, it doesn't go up. I don't know if there's a bit of a blockage or it's just the way my hand is.

His reply was, I'll make that decision. So, I said, well, you're just going to hurt me and put a needle in for no reason, so you might as well do it on the right.

We need to do it on the left. That was his answer. Okay.

When I say, he was talking to me like I'm a bit of shit, it may be an understatement.

If I wasn't in the position where I was relying on him, he would have got a mouthful, he puts in the line, it's all sweet but can't get no feedback from the drip no flow at all.

The machine that does the steady beeps, is not steady and beeps are not doing what the beeps are meant to be doing Blah, blah, blah, blah, blah. So, the lady, the young Filipino, said to him, you know, he told you that done all this yesterday, and he basically told her, shut up.

So now what we have is young nurse who's beside me, very pleasant, very helpful, very nice, very reassuring and part of a lovely team of people along with this man who's come in, who's obviously not part of their team, he's come in for the day, Who's horrible. So, someone says to him, can I talk to you in the other room? So, they go into the other room.

Now they're having a big row. Now imagine this. I'm lying there, my bollocks are hanging out. I'm scared, I'm nervous. Well, scared is nervous. I'm in a place that I've never been in before and I've got these people having a row about me.

They come out and it all starts again. this geezer hasn't changed his attitude. he's still horrible, talking to everyone like they're dirt. and it may just be his English, it may have been just the way he communicates, and he might have been an alright person, but the way he communicated with the English that he had was not very pleasant. So anyway, I'm in a position where they're trying to do what they've got to do.

He goes into my right hand, the drip goes in, everything is fine, and Just before I go out, they put the mask on for the air before anything is turned on.

Take some deep breaths and little tear runs down my face, runs out of my eye, down the back, past the mask, down to my ear and one of the other doctors in there said, is Mr Bates, okay? Is he sweating? the lady says, no, it's a tear.

I smiled at her and looked up and she said, I think he's very angry. and I just nodded. I was angry. then I was asleep.

When I woke up in recovery, I woke up in a way that I can only describe as being on a metal bed, wet, right, and it's plugged into the electric mains.

I have never felt anything like it. My legs were jumping.

The pain running up and down my spine was unbelievable.

My arms were jumping. It was like nothing I've ever experienced.

The pain and the jumping the kicking out it was just shocking. Excuse the pun.

It was a shock. It was shocking. This young neurosurgeon, I say young, I don't know how old he is, but he. He was younger than me, he comes to see me and, I am in so much pain that I can't even talk.

I'm gripping on to the side of the bed and he says, oh, well, the surgery went well, and I think we got everything.

I obviously said, you think you got everything? Then the obvious question to this absolutely prick of a man was, why have I woken up feeling like I'm sitting in an electric chair? what it is?

He replied that the spinal cord was so compressed and was just on the verge of rupture and its now decompressing, so your nerves are reacting in a way that it is.

The decompression of your system is making your nerves react in a strange way.

Your legs are going to jump uncontrollably, blah, blah, blah, blah, blah.

We will give you something for the pain.

I said, okay, fair enough, you believe what a neurosurgeon tells you.

Especially one that thinks that he walks on air and that he is god’s gift to humanity.

I get taken back up to the ward, and now I'm struggling, my legs are jumping like I've never seen before.

It's like someone's keeps hitting me with a cattle prod.

Bang, bang, bang, and you're thinking, how long does this go on for?

I go through the day of this cattle prod experience and loads and loads of painkiller, morphine and other meds.

The radiologist comes and sees me and he says, we've done really well.

We think we've got it, but I'm going to send you down for an MRI because it's the only way that we will know if we've got it.

Okay, fair enough.

I go down for an MRI in this hospital that was so, so, so, so professional and I mean that in an extremely sarcastic way.

They took me down to an MRI machine that was condemned and waiting to be taken out for a new one to be installed.

They take me in and there's a couple of young staff who will be doing the MRI.

I asked, what are you putting me in there for? It's clearly broken.

They said, no, it's not broken, it’s not condemned. It's being ripped out to for a new one to go in. It works.

So, I said, so you're going to get a proper MRI from this? and he said, oh, yeah, yeah, what it is, this is an urgent one. We can't fit you in in the other room where the new one is. So, we do this one here. So, okay, fair enough. So, I go in, I have my MRI, I go back upstairs. Now, this is Wednesday.

I've been in the hospital three days now, this is Wednesday. I go back up to the room and again they tell me once they look at the MRI, if they've got everything, then I'll be going home within the next couple of days if I could pee.

By now I can feel my legs again.

I can stand up. I can weight bare; I can stand up with a walking frame.

Things are looking good. It's better than it was before I went down.

So, you would think, they've done their job.

I sit there all-day Thursday, can't pee and I'm thinking, why don't they come up with the MRI results? So, the young nurses fit a catheter.

They empty me out, right? You're still not going home until you can pee.

I said, what do you mean going home? I've not seen this neurosurgeon and he said that if they've reached the fistula and completed a perfect seal exactly where it needs to be reached, then I can go home on Friday. If not, he'd be opening me up on Friday.

So, they said, oh, what he said is, because you're very heavy and you will have to lay on your stomach to do the surgery. He's very concerned about it.

So, the embolization is the way to go.

He doesn't think he's going to be doing the operation on Friday. So, I said, but does that mean he's got everything? and they said, oh, we don't know yet. You've got to talk to him.

Okay, fair enough.

I don't see him Thursday, and I don't see him Friday, as he was clearly floating around heaven speaking with God or bringing the dead back to life.

The radiologist comes around and sees me and by Friday, I can walk on the walker, and they send a physiotherapist round to see me. they say, if you can go up and down the stairs holding onto the handrail, you can go home.

So, I hold onto the handrail. I manage to get up and down the stairs. Bang. Friday is home time.

A friend comes and collects me. I can go home. And I told him I could pee, but I couldn't, so they let me home. I go home. Then the rest of the story starts.

A couple of weeks later I receive an email stating that the embolization was only a partial success and was incomplete.

The result of the embolization was improved but not resolved signal changes to the spinal cord, still some flow voids and a follow up angiogram to be carried out once settled.

Chapter 22: Dream Home

The Christmas, before the finding out of the fistula after knee surgery had been done long before my wife and I decided we were going to pack up and go and live in Germany.

We had our young son, Henry. We had been in a good position at work, both of us. My wife was an associate director, I was a senior project manager, but we were spending a lot of time getting to work in traffic.

London's not what it once was. things were changing at work and it was just a better off situation all round to move to Germany. So, my wife put in her notice and being in the position she was in, she had to give us six weeks' notice. So, our plans where she gives her notice in first week back at work in January. So that takes us around till June. I only had to give a month's notice, so I was going to give my notice in May. So, I get released from hospital and the dream is we go to Germany.

We live in and around the area of where my in laws live. both of my wife's parents are still alive and I will get myself a Harley Davidson and I can go out for rides on Sundays; I've got the freedom of the bike and my wife will be around her family, her friends that she grew up with, her best friends and we're going to bring our little son up in a different environment.

He's not going to be up in London or Essex or in, the places that I grew up.

So that's what we've decided.

I get an email from the doctor, and nonchalantly, in his arrogant way, the email reads that we had managed to reach a percentage of the fistulas, albeit one is not sealed, blah, blah, blah. But we'd like to see you again for an MRI in April, by now I'm walking again, so I think they've cured it.

I'm not having the weakness around the hips. I'm not feeling too bad. I think that I'm cured. we're preparing to go to Germany to live. The April date comes for the MRI, so I go in, I have my MRI and angiogram and miraculously the embolization had sealed itself and everything was good.

I have my appointment in the private hospital again in Brentwood with this neurosurgeon and I looked him in the eye and I said, right, are things going to get better? and he said, yes, things are going to get better. Now, I can't tell you how much better. I can't tell you whether you will fully recover, but nerves can take anything up to two years to realign themselves and the way you will be in two years' time is how you will be for the rest of your life. So, I said to him, well, I've got some amazing spasms, you know, I've got things that at night that I'm almost kicking the quilt off the bed.

He decided that he will get you in to see a nerve specialist and he will do a nerve conduction study right the way through, from the top of your head down to the end of your toes.

I have these pins put all over me, all these electrodes connected. and this nerve specialist says that the situation is the way nerves are and nerves can re realign themselves.

They can do this over a period of two years and during this time these uncontrollable spasms will sort themselves out, they will stop. And where you are in two years' time is what you will have for the rest of your life.

I come away from that, I see the neurosurgeon again and I say to him, look, I'm in a position with work if you think I'm going to be okay, then we will be emigrating to Germany, his reply was yep, yep, you've got no problems whatsoever. I will do a full report and we're quite happy to let you have it to take to a German doctor.

Okay, fine. So, all the drama is now finished and the next bit of anxiety is what comes with any house move but this one has the added stress as we are moving to Germany.

Our house is being sold; we've got to get all our timing right; we've got to make sure that the lawyers get us out of the house at the time that we can move to Germany.

We need to organize a company from Germany that will come and pack up the whole house and we can hand the keys over, walk away. We need to get rid of the Porsche, we need to get rid of the BMW. we need them sorted out. So, our drama now is the normal drama of emigrating to another country, not health issues. The health issues are gone; everything is fine as far as health is concerned and I'm walking again. So, the big day comes.

For two days, these German men are in the house packing up, boxing up. They had a lot of work to do.

We had a five-bedroom house, it was one of them five-bedroom houses that if you've got the space, we managed to fill it up.

No two ways about it. I like to buy a lot of crap; my wife is also the same. I think she's got shares in Amazon, but I've got this thing about Stone Island jackets, Sergio Tashina Fila Adidas trainers everywhere in boxes, you can imagine there's a lot of stuff to go.

So, the Porsche has gone, that's been collected, we're down to one car.

We got the BMW. when the Porsche was taken away, it was my wife's car, but I come from a council estate in North London. I never thought I'd be driving a Porsche.

So, when the man came and collected it and drove off in it, I just felt sick, sick inside when that car disappeared down the road.

Next couple of days pass, the BMW goes and we're off.

We've got a Nissan Qashqai, we're off, we're going to Germany. So, the lorry departs, we hand the keys in, we get in the car and we leave.

Henry in the back. Henry's a three-year-old, my three-year-old son is going to brought up as a GERMAN.

Our new life in Germany is about to start. we've got our rental apartment; we bought a plot of land three years prior just in case we ever moved to Germany. it's a nice plot on a hill surrounded by trees, try to imagine where we live in Germany it is a small town, we live in a small village and it's high up in the hills at the highest point of the area and we are surrounded by pine trees.

You really don't have to go far to, feel like you're driving on a street in Switzerland or driving on a road in Canada or whatever. There are some amazing places to drive around there and for me being a history buff, there's the story of Arminius Herman the German, this is the area in the Teutoburger Forest where I live, which is one hundred fifty-six kilometres long, where twenty thousand Romans were defeated by the Germans, it was their single biggest defeat in Roman history when they tried to take on the Germanic tribes.

Arminius was the son of a Cherusci leader who was taken hostage by the Romans with his brother Flavus,

What they used to do was take the sons of the tribal leaders so the tribal leaders would never rise up against the Romans. So, the sons would end up being trained and they would live as Romans.

They knew how to fight, they soon rose through the ranks became high ranking soldiers, but what happened, Arminius had different ideas when he came back, instead of coming back as a Roman, he come back and he united the tribes and the tribes stood against the Romans. So, where the monument for Arminius stands right at the top of the highest point in this area, which, again, is up a big, big country road full of pine trees and is absolutely beautiful.

So, we've got this plot of land on the hill. I'm thinking, as soon as that house is built, I'm getting my Harley.

All I could think of, I am getting my Harley Davidson with the last ten grand.

So, we start making the plans, Bee is dealing with the drawings, with the architects, we've got the builder on board, but the house, like I said, is on a hill. and I'm now getting worse.

I've gone from being able to walk to everything coming back again.

Are there more fistulas? If they come back, what's happening to me? So, I make an appointment with a German neurologist, and this man is supposedly the best.

When I say supposedly, I don't mean that as a negative, people told us he was one of the best, a Hungarian doctor that has runs a department in one of the big hospitals in Paderborn.

We go in and see him, we've got all of the files, we've got all of the MRIs.

We explain the story and just with the explanation. He looks at me and says, sounds like you've had an infarction in your back, which is basically a stroke in my spinal cord.

He looks at the MRI and his conclusion was that my spinal cord has had a stroke and I've got to basically take, vitamin B12 with this and that to help with the nerves, and there's not a lot anyone can do, but if they could, he would and he promised that he would do everything within his power to help, So, I come away from there thinking, oh, wow, he's a really, really good doctor and may possibly be able to help.

He's going to cure me; he's going to solve it. Well, that was the first bit of hope that was dashed because he wasn't actually going to do anything. He was very distant; he was hard to get hold of and he was private and we could not afford to put the thousands and thousands and thousands into this doctor.

We go back to the property where, we've worked out the kitchen, we've got a big double garage that's going to have a balcony over the top. we're going to use the roof with glass panelling around it. This house is going to be wonderful, as you look at it from the street, it looks like it's two stories.

So, there would be the kitchen, the living level. You go upstairs, you've got the main bedroom, Henry's bedroom, a bathroom and then what you've got in the roof is a total playroom for Henry with a ladder going up to was going to be out of this world.

The house would be on three levels, full of stairs with a garden on a hill.

Where Henry's and my play room was going to possibly, was in the basement and I was going to go back to breeding my beloved Dogue de Bordeaux.

I was going to have a puppy whelping room, a big sofa with the big screen up, we was going to have a room with some weights in it for a gym and our peloton bike.

There would be big double glazed open windows that constantia backwards and forwards looking out over the hill that we're built into. But the hill was now a massive problem as we'd have to cut steps down to the next level of the garden, then again down to the next level of the garden, but I'm getting worse.

So, I go to my local doctor who's looked at my files, we laugh and joke because the file is as thick as a telephone book, but I have struck gold with my doctor he is an Anglophile.

He travels to London twice a year, he's worked in England.

He is the most perfect doctor for me because number one, he gives me time, number two, he cares and number three, he's just a fantastic person. So, I go to see him and he says to me, there's a hospital down in Bad Wildungen called the Werner-Wicker-Klinik that specializes in spinal cords injuries.

It's the best hospital you can imagine.

I'm going to write a letter. We're going to get you appointment and we're going to get you down there and they will sort you out.

I get my appointment, it was on a Monday, so on the Sunday I've booked a hotel and I go down there, I'm in the hotel, a bit anxious, thinking about what's going to happen.

The day comes, and I must say that I've never in the time that I've lived here had any real issues with not being able to speak German, and you've got to imagine that by now I'm on tablets for epilepsy, I'm on tablets for MS, I'm on tablets for Parkinson's disease and all of these tablets are trying to control the signals that I'm losing in my spinal cord down to my legs, and up from my legs to my brain. I'm on gabapentin, which is a horrible drug in my opinion, that makes my mind fuzzy and my balance is not so good, things are not going so well at this stage, but I'm at this super-duper hospital that's got the doctors that are going help me, they will do something, even if they have to do the opening my back and I have a two year recovery period, they are going to make me better.

There's always this hope dies last theory and these people are my last hope.

In the hospital I can't find anyone who's going to speak English to me, which is not their fault, it's mine and with all this medication, me trying to learn German is nigh on impossible, all I can ask for is a cup of coffee, a beer or a couple of beers or a cake, that's all I've learned.

I get to the waiting room; I'm sitting there incredibly anxious.

The doctor comes out to see me, we go in, he's read the letter, he's read my file, sends me off for an X ray, calls me back in and he calls his boss in.

I've got another professor sitting there and they have said there's nothing they can do.

They say that it's all down to the nerves having to repair themselves and although you feel that you're getting worse, this is part of the recovery process and it's going to take a while but you know, there's nothing they can surgically do for me.

So, I come away and I'm devastated and it just so happens that when I come away on the way back if with a seventeen-kilometre detour, there's a place called the Eder Dam, this is one of the dams that was demolished, destroyed by the British RAF during the dam buster sequence of destruction in the dams in the Ruhr valley.

I thought I would go there for a coffee, I just needed to be alone. I wanted to be on my own as I've had enough by now, I'd really have had enough.

Every time I got sent to a hospital, every time I went somewhere, I never got any good news, nothing was good, nothing that anyone was telling me was a positive so, oh, what's going to be, what it's going to be.

If after two years of nerve repairing itself that's how you are, that's what you're going to be stuck with. So, I go to the Eder dam, I grab myself a coffee and I look at the dam and I think, yep, this is it. This is perfect. Absolutely perfect. The wall's not too high for me to get over and the drop is absolutely massive.

My decision was made, it wasn't to kill myself on that day.

It was a preferred place of suicide decision; this is the place in Germany where I decided that I would take my own life.

If I keep getting this bad news and I keep getting given hope, that dies and the rugs that are constantly pulled away from under my feet.

This is the place that I would end it because there's no way you could survive that drop.

I stood there for maybe an hour, hour and a half, and I think even the tourists that were walking up and down, must have been wondering why I was planted in the same spot looking at the drop and not the water.

You can walk the, the length of the dam up to the other side and back again and I was still there.

They were looking at me and probably thinking, he's been there for an hour.

I was just staring down, looking at where I would land.

At first you think, would I survive that? Could you? Because you could roll. This dam is at a bit of an angle. Would you roll all the way down and then just hit the bottom with less impact than if it was a sheer drop.

You're now analysing the whole situation, but I came away thinking that is the place that I'm going to do myself.

I walked back to the car. Well, I limped back to the car with my crutches and I am thinking, Yeah, that's the number one spot.

I'm driving back and now I seem to be quite euphoric and jubilant; I've actually found somewhere that I could end it, this has not turned out too bad a day after all

Although the doctors can't do nothing for me. I'm not going to live like this. I'm totally refusing to live like this.

So, if I get worse, that's where I'm going to do it.

I'm driving back and I go over this absolutely massive bridge. It's absolutely huge, and I look and I think, right, this is better, this place and that fence, I could get over it, but you know what? There was grass all underneath It. It was a valley. It was a valley of grass, and I tell you what, I will be fucked if I am jumping onto grass because knowing my luck, I won't fucking die, I would end up jumping when it's been a rainstorm the night before and it's all soggy and I just land in the mud, make a great big dent and nothing happens to me. I just end up with a headache or a broken leg.

So, I dismissed that one, but it wasn't long before I reached another bridge that's got a nice wide asphalted or concreted road underneath.

The barriers are not too high, this was the place, the actual place.

I could de risk doing it at the dam.

There's lots and lots of tourists that would see me go, so I'd have to do it at night, but this bridge on the way back from the dam, I think was even better. So, I've had a good look at this and it is even better. So, I drive home. I've known I've got a plan.

I've got my English plan and I've got my German plan and the English plan is a very, very good one because what I could do, is go over to England, see my son Luc, who's now twenty-nine. I could be driving back to the ferry port. I can get to the piece of road where it's seventy miles per hour and there's no barriers in the middle, where all of the foreign articulated lorries are coming up the road, up the hill and doing seventy mile an hour. When they get off the hill, they come onto the A2 near Whitfield roundabout, they pick up speed. I will make out I'm writing a text, I throw the phone down into the footwell, I drive head on, straight into a lorry. Bang. Dead.

Now that looks like I've not killed myself. So now we're getting to the stage where if you jump off the Eder dam, deliberate, if you jump off of the bridge, deliberate, if you're driving home from seeing your son for the last time and you drive into a lorry but you've dropped, thrown your phone into the footwell and it looks like you've lent over to get your phone and then you drive into the lorry and you're dead. Right, sorted. It's not your fault, is it? It's not your fault. But either way, I'm now of the opinion that any more bad news, any sadness that hits me, I will be taking one of the options because I can't go on with this. So, I'm happy now. I know how I am going to go. I know how I'm going to end it, when I choose to.

DECISION MADE.

Chapter 23: Stalag

It was becoming very clear that this dream home that we were going to build on the hill was really just a dream. the house wasn't just on a hill going upwards when you drove up to the road, it was on a hill going down over three levels of garden. It was going to be three floors in the house, so lots of stairs.

When you come out the garage, there was going to be quite a severe ramp.

So, we had to make the heartbreaking decision that as my health was declining and my ability to walk was getting worse, we've had several doctors, specialists and neurosurgeons say that the way you'll be in two years is the way you'll be for life and I was only by this stage, eight months in and getting worse. There were no improvements at all.

It was a resoundingly getting worse, that there was no point building this house.

So, we were now having to look for an apartment, a rental apartment so we could move into while we looked for another house that fitted our needs.

Now remember that we had spent a good chunk of our money on a plot of land.

We were now in a bit of a situation where I had broken my wife's heart, which she would never say but I had or accept it.

I was carrying the burden of disappointing Bee and the money that was invested in the land come from her.

I was every night and every day carrying that burden of what I had done to her because it's all my fault that I can't go for a walk with my son. It's all my fault I can't ride a push bike with my son. It's all my fault that we could not build the house the dream home.

She can't have her dream kitchen. the burdens I was carrying mentally were becoming more and more to the forefront of my thought process.

I couldn't think of anything positive.

Everything I thought about was negative everything was my fault. By now my toes had started to bend and on my right foot and my right foot had started to drop.

So, I had the classic foot drop where I was walking along, tripping over and I was doing my best. I was falling over and I was hurting myself and it just wasn't working for us.

We found this bungalow, a massive place.

We went into the bungalow; it was an old people's house and it was completely unfinished.

They had run out of money.

They had finished the downstairs to a really poor standard.

The upstairs was just a few rooms, of block work, walls just really, really unfinished.

The insulation was in, but just joists. it was awful.

We came away, we had a good think, we put an offer in.

After a bit of negotiating, we managed to buy the house.

We spent a year doing this house up, we gutted it, moved walls, ripped out two bathrooms to make one big one and give us more bedroom space, we even sank the bath into the ground so that I would be able to get into it, even though we need the fire brigade to get me out of it.

We now have what we believe is to be the perfect house for us. It's a bungalow for me.

So, I sleep downstairs, bathrooms downstairs. but we've also got the upstairs.

We've got an office; we've got a suite bedroom and a bathroom for visitors.

We've got a massive playroom which has got my 70-inch TV.

It's good for Henry's, all his toys, it's worked out really, really well, we've got space for the dogs.

Everything has worked out well, but it comes with a price.

We've got outstanding debt now and we've got a plot of land that my wife sunk her money into that hasn't sold, two years later and that burden again is on my mind.

This burden of finance now is on my mind, any setback, anything that comes becomes my burden literally anything.

As I'm writing this now, the weathers bad. We live in a place where it snows. I can't go and get my son from school because if I don't walk good enough to get my son from school because it's on a hill and there could be snow, there could be ice.

Well, I know there's snow, I refuse to use my crutch when I go to his school because I don't want him to be ashamed of me, so my wife has to do it. So, it's like she's got two children, that is another mental burden.

Even my son knows now that if I fall, just ask some questions. Are you alright, dad?

Do you want me to do anything? Do you need me to help you get up? Blah, blah, blah.

These are the things I live with.

I get to my doctors and I tell him that I'm falling over all the time.

He looks in his book and he come up with a prescription for a foot brace.

I get measured up for this foot brace. It's a carbon foot brace that does this, does that, blah, blah, blah and now I've got not only a crutch, but I'm now wearing a leg brace and with the leg brace comes the humiliation of being what I believe to be a youngish man in my mid to late fifties but carrying this overwhelming feeling of humiliation, I feel embarrassed, I can't do what I want to do. I'm walking with a crutch. I've now got a leg brace on and low and behold, I can't hold my wee.

So, I'm either pissing myself or my bladder is getting so full up that it is feels like it's going to burst.

Once again, I get taken into hospital and I have to have a catheter bag.

Things are getting worse, It's a downward spiral now.

My doctor says, I'm going to send you to a neurological professor in Detmold.

I go and see this professor.

He has never experienced the SDAVF and decides to admit me into his hospital.

I sit in his hospital for ten days.

It's a neurological wing, so. Neurological means It's your brain.

I sit there with people screaming for their mums and when I say screaming for their mums, I mean every waking hour.

These people could be in their eighties or nineties but still want their mums.

There are people in my room shitting themselves.

There are men arguing over people snoring. It was horrendous. Honestly, it was what I imagine prison to be like but without the smells and with me thinking that I am as funny fuck, I was doing a little thing on Facebook, a daily diary like I was in Coldit prisoner of war camp.

I checked in as:

Prisoner Bates

Stalag Klinik Nova

Bad Salzlufen

Station 14

Cell 118

I was trying to make it into a joke the way I do, but things were hard.

You're in this situation in a room, and you are no farther away than eight hundred millimetres from the next bed. There are no curtains, you're sharing a bathroom with people. It was just shocking, and I ended up staying in this hospital for ten days and after another MRI, (I am surprised that I am not like Homer Simpson with all that radiation).

One day one of the doctors come to me and was struggling a little bit in English and I asked her to call and speak with my wife, Bianca, and it was agreed that a professor near Dortmund would take me and do what they could with regard to this fistula.

The local Professor had exhausted all options with regard to how to treat me.

I'm now on the fourth professor. So again, I've just done ten nights in this hospital in a neurological ward. They're going to put me in a taxi, send me off for two hours to a place where it's too far for my wife to visit and I'm going to be there alone, not knowing what people are doing but they're going to fix me.

Theres that word **HOPE** again, this word hope is a killer. Hope is absolutely soul destroying. It messes with your brain in a way that is indescribable.

I'm in this taxi and I go to this new hospital and I get myself settled in and the first day I am sitting in a reception area.

I'm talking to Bianca as my phone is working fine because I'm in the reception area and it keeps me out of the room.

I get up and I think, oh, I might need to go to the toilet.

I walk back to the toilets, as I'm walking along, I can feel my legs wet and I look behind me and there is just a trail of shit, like you've dragged a dead body and the bloods on the floor, there was just a trail of diarrhoea all behind me.

I get into the toilet; I pull the red emergency cord.

The young nurse comes to me and I'm just standing there crying, saying, I'm sorry. I'm so sorry. I'm really in a mess, not to mention the floors.

It was just unbelievable and I was finding it really, really hard to cope.

I have no control of my bowel; I've got no control of my bladder that either let's go or fills up. I'm now clearly losing control of my bodily functions and it's become really difficult. So, while I'm in this hospital, I get taken down for an angiogram or angiograph as it's called in Germany.

I go down there and the normal thing, you're lying there, you've got your paper knickers on, you're looking at the lights as they dragging you all through this hospital.

You go down. It's like I said earlier, it's different in Germany.

Over here they take you in, in your bed. It stays in a certain area.

Then they say, can you get on here? So, you climb up and you get on this other bed and they take you in and people are chatting and it's all very nice, but you're in the operating theatre, which gives you a level of anxiety.

No matter who you are, no matter how tough you think you are, there's a level of anxiety. It's always better to be in a separate room they put you to sleep you don't go in and see all the tools laying out. You don't go in and see all these big lights and machines and, you've not got all the beeping going, so it's always nicer to not have to go through that. But anyway, I had the angiogram.

I Wake up in recovery, but I'm bad, so they put me in a critical unit area. My breathing was bad. I've never been like this after surgery, but I was in a room on my own.

I had every machine on me. I had a nurse come in every couple of minutes, I was very bad and I was scared.

The fear was because normally I wake up from surgery as if I've not had surgery. I'm very, very lucky but on this particular occasion, to wake up with all these machines on you and you're struggling, you feel really, really bad, I was only like that for a matter of hours. Don't get me wrong, it was just a matter of hours. But by the next morning, the doctor came in to see me and she said, look, we've found a gap in the embolization and that could possibly be causing all these problems. So, I said, but they told me that it had sealed in April.

I've got an email from the doctor in England telling me that it had completed the embolization.

My head was fucking spinning, those wankers in England when I had the April angiogram said that it had managed to seal itself. She said, well, I can tell you it's not sealed itself and that's what we need to do tomorrow.

So, I said, yeah, fine, yeah, no worries and then do you reckon I'll start getting better?

So, she said, well, we hope so, let's get it done.

The following morning comes, and I am ready for my surgery.

Only this time, I am ready to give up, I start thinking about waking up in a bad way the day before, it clearly couldn’t have been that bad as they were going to do the same again today, this time I was praying.

DEAR LORD, I AM NOT A RELIGIOUS MAN, BUT COULD YOU SEE YOUR WAY TO TAKING ME TODAY.

I HAVE HAD ENOUGH AND I DON'T WANT TO WAKE UP.

They put me on my bed. you go through, like in the films, you're looking at the lights as you're going all down through all these corridors. You're plonked into this operating area; you're put onto the operating table. A man comes over, pulls off my paper knickers, my little winkle is hanging out, my bollocks are sitting there clear for everyone to see and then I hear shouting in the background and I'm thinking, this is Deja vu.

I've had all this before in England with people shouting in the background.

It turned out that I had signed paperwork for the very first angiogram. No one had put any paperwork in front of me for the second and as I'd not signed any paperwork, I couldn't have this embolization done.

I laid on this bed for a good forty minutes with my bollocks hanging out. Embarrassed, humiliated, ashamed, while I'm listening to all these people in the background, they're calling other people, they're calling other doctors, they're calling the boss, they're trying to get round it, obviously, but not telling me anything, as it turns out in the end, they didn't do it.

So, I had all of the process of going down in an operating theatre, laying on the table, all the lights were on me, the drip was on me, everything was ready to go, So I said, give me the piece of paper, I'll sign it now. Nope, it has to be twenty-four hours.

So, they gave me the bit of paper. While I was laying on the table, I signed the piece of paper, they pulled my blanket down so my balls couldn't be seen, dragged me back up to the room, and that was it for another twenty-four hours. So, the anxious wait started again.

Next morning, I go down, I'm having my surgery done. I go down normal, everything is fine. Don't even want to go into detail for the book. You've heard it all before, lines in this, that, this, that, blah, blah, blah, wake up, everything's fine. Did you get to the bit that was left by the surgeons in England? Yes, it's all done. Will I get better? Yes, we hope so.

Can't guarantee anything, but we've gone as far as we can go.

So, I respond with the obligatory Okay.

I stay in hospital for another couple of days, then I'm released. They put me in a taxi, two hours home, life is going to get better.

I wrote to the hospital near Dortmund and asked about failure of glue and as it prone to failure, can’t they open me up and scrape it out, I was obviously desperate and pissing in the wind.

I received the life changing reply in the January.

The letter stated that they could not remove the glue as I had suggested and that the continued problems that I was having was due to the stroke that I had in my spinal cord caused by an overuse of glue used in the UK at the first embolization. WHAT!!!!!!!!

There we have it.

Within a few days of receiving that letter, my head started to feel better.

I had to get used to the new me, the new normal.

Bollocks to all that hope rubbish, let’s move along now

.

Chapter 24: Leave Me Alone

I got some really good friends, Robbie and Tracy.

Robbie's Jamaican, bred, born in England, but bred from Jamaican parents. And that means that Robbie will be late for everything. He will book a flight when he's ready to, but we talk about it for weeks and weeks. Finally, I got the date when Robbie and Tracy were coming to visit. Now, you would not believe how happy I am that they are coming to visit.

I go and get them from the airport. So excited. They come, get them in the house. We have some food, we have some drinks, stay up late. Really, really lovely evening. The next day we're going to go into town. We're going to go down to Paderborn.

It's nice and brisk. It's cold, big coats on scarves. Really, really looking forward to a nice day. So, we get them in the car, everyone's wrapped up, ready to go and I forgot to pick something up indoors, I can't remember what it was maybe a selfie stick or something like that so we could get pictures of all of us together. I walk in the house, bang. I've gone over. Not only have I gone over, I've now cracked some ribs because I've landed on my elbow and the ribs have gone. I knew I cracked ribs. I heard my ribs go.

Robbie and my wife come running into the house. They know something had happened. You could hear the bang. I mean, I'm a heavy man. You could probably have heard the bang in Berlin.

I'm lying there and Robbie tries to help me up and I get angry. Leave me alone. Leave now.

I'm ashamed. I'm. I've fallen over. I'm like a kid. So, Robbie wants to help. Robbie, leave me alone. Leave me alone. Robbie. Don't touch me. Now he's upset and he's wondering why I'm acting like this. What people don't understand is I have to lay there and work out if anything's damaged to me.

I've got two new knees, two metal knees and still can't safely walk, I've cracked some ribs, so they help me up once I've realized that I'm all right. The rib situation, when you crack ribs, they are not so bad at the time but the pain really comes later on. I know what was going to come on later. I know how bad I was going to be. So, we get to the car. Are you all, right? You sure you want to go? You sure you want to go? Yeah, yeah, of course I do. Of course I do. Now I'm not ruining this trip. This trip that I've looked forward for them coming for ages and ages and ages. I was so excited. And now I've fallen over and it made me feel sick.

Sick that I can't even have my friends come to visit. So we go to town, we have a lovely day. Over the period of the next few days, ribs start really, really doing what I knew they were going to do. They start really, really hurting. But I've got to put on a brave face.

I've got to hide from them that I'm in absolute agony. I am in bits and I've got to hide it. So, everyone stays up a little bit late on the Saturday night and Robbie and Tracy are going home on Sunday. So about 10pm. I take Henry to bed and then I say, look, I'm really tired, I have to go. I could not hide it anymore. I had to go to bed and leave Bianca with them and they had a nice evening. But the sad thing is I didn't have a nice evening. So that's the sort of thing I have to live with.

The falling over, The breaking things, the ribs, the elbows, the shoulders etcetera.

All of these incidents of looking forward to friends coming over then a fall, or playing with my little boy and falling over, or shitting myself at Lucs place etc, fuck with my and send me spiralling in a new depression, and once the spiral starts, it's like a tornado, its sucks everything upwards.

Chapter 25: Lokomat

During this whole period of hell, I had reached the stage of being totally immobile un-aided.

Physiotherapy wasn't doing anything and it was decided that I had reached the stage where I had to have sessions on a Loko mat robotic rehabilitation machine.

I could still drive, I was wearing nappies, I needed a pair of crutches, I carried a bag everywhere I go, it contained nappies, clean pants, clean t-shirt and trousers, doggy poo bags and rubber gloves.

I walk into this room and see this state-of-the-art walking machine and it was truly fascinating.

You stand on a treadmill, the therapist straps you in to a harness, and then straps sensors and motors to your thighs and calves and then lift you up in the air so that you are not weight baring at all.

The idea is that this machine teaches you how to walk, to correct your gait and allow your muscle to learn how to walk again.

If you work to hard, the machine gets pissed off with you, if you don't work hard enough, the machine gets pissed off with you so the idea is that you do exactly what the robot wants you to do and you are trying to keep steady by following a smiley or sad emoji face.

When I started with the Lokomat, it was doing 80% of the work, so I had total spasticity in my legs and only 20% function.

After my first session, I was alive, I was buzzing, I almost skipped out to the car and drove home on the phone to Bee to telling her that this was it, this was going to give some life back.

Well fuck me, the next morning, I felt like I had run the London marathon after climbing Everest before swimming the Atlantic.

I didn't feel like that for a day, it was pretty much a week, I probably felt a bit better just as the next session was due.

See what happens with my condition is that I can't get stronger, but I can very easily get weaker, so I have to maintain what I have as best I can, the blood flow doesn't do what it needs to or reach the important parts that require it.

Over the next few months, I start to see improvements, and by the time that I was signed off from the Lokomat I was as good as I could get and I was doing 80% of the work with 20% robot power.

The therapist even brought a football in was holding in front of me to get me to use force to try and kick it.

It was amazing, I was feeling a bit happier but still had falls and relapses and was still incontinent.

Chapter 26: Universal Medical Centre Groningen

As my visceral organs are failing me and everything from the nipple line down seems to be giving up, starting first with the Bladder, prostate, bowels, colon.

I have neurological bowel disorder issue where it's not doing what it's meant to be doing.

It's going really slow and then building up with constipation. Not going to toilet for a few days and then literally you get a lump come out and then like a jet washer. So, this will run down your legs, up your back, you'll have it in your hair, it just zaps the life out here.

I was referred to a local doctor. Very, very good, lovely woman, really nice.

Go in now, sits me in a chair, says take your pants off, spins me round and boom, fingers straight in and she's saying, squeeze.

I want to see how good your sphincter can squeeze onto things.

Go on, squeeze, squeeze really hard and believe me when I say that I have never felt so humiliated in all my life, even with all that I have been through.

So, I'm trying to crack jokes and doing what I do with a finger up my bum, luckily, she is a tiny little woman.

They put me at ease by saying, the thing is, we do this for a living. the next person who comes in, and the one who comes in after that, we're seeing this all day long, we don't think nothing of it, so try and relax and they reassured me that the next time I come in and the time after that, it will be less mentally traumatic and I will feel a lot better about it.

I said, oh, you are planning on doing this regular then? we had a good joke, but the top and bottom of it was they offered me a pacemaker.

The pacemaker goes into your back and then is connected by a probe to a nerve in your spinal cord that goes down to your sphincter.

It's controlling my backside.

It's controlled by a Samsung Galaxy, oddly enough, you put this credit card sized sensor over the monitor in your back, you go onto your phone, you press the button, eight, nine, ten, eleven, what you want it to be to control your sphincter so you shouldn't be pooing everywhere.

Another operation. and by now I'm done, I'm really, really done. I've had enough. and going back to earlier pages, when I said that I was quite happy for the hospital to make a mistake. I was in the same frame of mind again.

If a mistake was made, my sons couldn't blame me, my wife couldn't blame me, I was in the clear then I'd gone off to the next life which, sadly I don't believe there is one. It'd be nice if I thought there was because I'd be even more comfortable with it but I'm now going into hospital, going to be pulled around again, wake up with a monitor in my back and I am going to control everything via this Samsung Galaxy. I'm going to turn it up, turn it down, do what I want with it and life's good.

Another operation, same old, same old. I'm not going to go into that. The detail of the looking at lights as you wheel down and pulling your pants off, etc have the operation done. Two weeks later, I'm fine, good as gold. Nonetheless, this implant did not do a thing. Imagine sitting on an electric current and when I say electric sitting on, I mean right in your tea tail holder. So, you turn it up and you can feel it going up and you're like whoa, whoa. But you get used to it very quickly now I've got it really as high as I can handle it.

So, I get this done. I am still wearing nappies; I can only half empty the bladder. So, I still have periods of real bad infections of which one of them was when I was working in Holland.

I went out for a drink with the boys.

I was a Construction Director so never really accepted these invites, but this Saturday night, I accepted and went out for a drink with the boys, got mangled the way you do, absolutely spanned.

Had a real good night, good laugh, get in a cab back home to this nice little apartment I had.

Can't pee.

All through the night I'm getting up, sitting down, getting up, sitting down, I can't pee.

This goes right the way around till Monday. Now when you look at my stomach on the Monday, it looked like there was a football inside my stomach. It was so painful and what it did was give me an infection. So, I've now as rough as fuck.

I ring my governor up, say look, I can't come to work, I'm in a bad way and the first thing he says is you get to the hospital. I said, yeah, yeah, of course I will, yeah, yeah, no worries. I didn't. But I tell you what, when I had that infection, I was laying in this apartment on my own away from my family who were hundreds of miles away and I thought to myself, if this is it, what a horrible way to go.

Considering I would have accepted death on a hospital stretcher, I couldn’t handle dying alone in Holland soaked in my own piss.

I know that my visceral organs are going to pack up, but I weren't expecting them to pack up so soon.

Not after getting diagnosed and all that stuff. I wanted to do another ten, fifteen years, if I live till, I'm seventy-five, I weren't expecting to get there anyway. So, if I get there with this, it's all going to be ok, that's a good age.

I'm lying in this bed, I'm sweating, one minute I'm throwing the quilt off me, next minute I'm putting the quilt on me. Then in the night, when I did get some sleep and relaxed, a little bit of wee come out. So, I've now wet the bed in a place that's rented out, so that's not great.

My colleague Buck comes and collects me, gets me in the car and we are off to the hospital, they can see how much pain I'm in because I can't even stand up straight. It looks like I've got a bad back.

So, I get in now and this young nurse is chatting away, again a nice polite and conscientious young man, he says, right, I'll get this out of here, but what I got to do, I've got to take some bloods and we get some, a urine sample done for bacteria. So, I'm going to put you in, in one of the rooms, they take me down to this room and I'll tell you what, this hospital was like the fucking Hilton. It was absolutely unbelievable. You didn't queue for hours to get in.

They were nice, no one was rude. You just handed over your insurance card and sit there and wait in a nice stress-free environment.

Not like the casualty at the Whittington at the Archway.

This man says to me, look, I'm sorry, we're quite busy but we get these, these urine tests done as these bacterial samples done as soon as we can but they take quite a while because we don't know what you got in there.

I'm laying now and I'm pretty chilled. Young Buck goes out for his Christmas dinner with his governor and then comes back and I tell him that he didn't have to do this.

I'm safe in the hospital, I can get a sherbet home. Anyway, as a really lovely bloke. Good, old South African boy.

I'm sitting in the hospital, young doctor comes in to see me, asking me all the questions. I tell him about visceral organ starting to fail, bladder being the first told him I've got the pacemaker in the back and I must wear the nappies, etc, etc. they said, are you prone to infections? I replied oh yeah, I get them bad. But this one's been the worst. So must have been two or three hours. later she comes back in and she says, you've not only got one bacteria, but you've also got two bacteria in your bladder and a blood infection, the bacteria in your blood is why you thought you were on your way out. But what we're going to do, we're going to give you this tablet which is like Agent Orange.

My new best mate the GP said It's one of them things that either cures you or kills you.

So I was given this, I stayed until late that night, I was packed off home and over the next few days, I slowly but surely got better but another problem they found was when they were putting tubes in me, my, my prostate was a decent size, nothing wrong with it, done all the PSA tests and all that good stuff, but it was a little bit big at this time I must have been fifty seven, fifty eight. So go in and see a urologist. What's he wants to do? He wants to either Aqua Blast it, where that's taking chunks of it off, which means you could be constantly leaking or having to wear pads, etcetera. Or he can do the Urolift. Not Euro lift as in Euro, but as in urology. So, he's going to do this lift. I go in another surgery, I think I'm up to like twelve, thirteen at this stage and by now I'm thinking please just go sleep.

I keep waking up, I keep fucking waking up from these surgeries. You would not believe how disappointed I am to Keep waking up. So, he's done all these clips, I can't piss any better. So, I'm now in a position where I've got the choice of walking around with bags stuck to me legs or I learn how to self-catheterize. So I,

I start the task of self-catheterization which was absolutely scaring the life out of me because every time I've had a catheter, most of the times I was asleep and when I had had a catheter put in, in hospitals or by my doctor, I've always like held someone's hand and it's always, I've always had it in my brain, that this is going to be a killer, plus a lot of the time when people were forcing it in, they were, they were trying to force it in past the prostate that was being like Tony Adams in defence, it didn't want to let anything past it.

I start self-catheterizing. I'm back to normal now I'm running around out on the piss again at work. one story when I was on the town in Groningen, I walk in this toilet and there's a toilet and a urinal in the same room. So, no privacy, you know, typical European and I'm standing there and I'm like Robin Hood. Everywhere I go, I carry a bag. My bag has got fresh T shirt, fresh pants, wet wipes, dry wipes, dog poo bags, catheters, etcetera. Etc. So imagine being like Robin Hood. I've got my backpack on and it's. Instead of it being arrows that I pull out, I've got 300mm long catheters tubes that I'm getting ready to shove up my japs eye and there's a Dutch geezer having a piss in your urinal.

He is intrigued as I've got this thing out and he looked at me, so what are you doing? So, I said, sorry, mate, I don't speak Dutch. And he said, okay, in perfect English, the way they do. What are you doing? So, I said, I've got to put this in, get it past the prostate into the bladder, because my bladder's packed up, it doesn't work. He went, oh, you're joking. So no, no. So, he said, can I watch? of course you can. You're mad. As he's bending down to have a look at me threading this tube in my winkle, his pal comes in and his pal said to him, what are you doing? So, he said, come and have a look at this. I've got two geezers either side of me bending down looking at my winkle while I'm threading a tube straight in. As I get it in, it's catching a little bit. It's not, it's bending. It's not going quite to plan like usual when no one's watching, it flies in, but it's not going to plan on this occasion.

I get it, fiddle it, twist it round, bang, it goes in, piss comes out all into the toilet. These two Dutch bods go, YESSSSSSS and it's almost like Holland had just scored the winning goal in the World Cup final.

After celebrating that it had come out. we went outside, the toilet started, they started chatting to me, what's happened to you? So, I explained spinal cord stroke, blah blah, blah. I never had to buy a drink again that night. They were calling me a hero, a warrior. How can you live like that and still come out on the piss? Most people would give up, you know, I'm not going to give up. I won't. So, you know, that was one of the funny little ones. But learning to live with the pooing yourself and everything else, it starts zapping your confidence after a while. And I'm someone who wants a career in public speaking. I'm not quiet, I go into an office. I was in a level in the last project where I think there was one hundred people in the office that were below me with four, five, six hundred out on site. So, I'm not shy, I talk to the people at some of the biggest companies in the world, I never have an issue with things like that. But I'm now feeling my confidence being eroded.

I had a bit of an incident where a motor hit me in Germany and because I hadn't changed my license to a German one, they stopped me from driving for a few months, which meant every time I went backwards and forwards to Holland, I had to get a train and it was a six-hour one way trip on trains where when you go on smaller trains, the toilets are always locked and when I say locked it’s the red tape damaged and locked.

Then you're sitting there getting more and more anxious and I think a lot, a lot of the pooing yourself is anxiety, your body reacting to how your brain's feeling.

It was kind of, it was just becoming so unpleasant But you, you roll with it. This is, this is your new life, you are taking anti diarrhoea tablets every day. You're taking psyllium husk, you're doing all this researching as much as you can about natural remedies so you can have a decent, healthy, solid poo.

At this time, I didn't know that I had the neurogenic bowel disorder which was caused by the colon just slowing down that much that it just would not push the poo out. And it was, like I said earlier, it would get to the stage where it was stuck. You'd get a toxic build up behind it that would flush that lump out. Once that lump come out, you. It was deadly. And when I say deadly, it was. It was toxic. It would burn you. It was horrible.

This is my new life, where things are steadily getting worse and worse.

It isn't just about hospitals and being able to walk and balance, I've now got tubes to pee. I now where nappies.

If I can have a pee, it's half a pee, and then you're dribbling into your nappy.

Life's incredibly, hard. And with all this going on, I've got the urologist who calls me back and he says, you know, I think we're going to have to aqua blast you.

They blast the prostate and get a bit of it out. I don't know whether these clips are much good. I said, well, you did them. So, by now I'd had enough of surgeries. I've booked a private, Two hundred twenty euros a night for this private room. Getting there on the day of the surgery and it's fucking handsome, really nice.

I'm sitting there, no one comes in and sees me.

Ten o', clock, eleven o', clock, twelve o', clock, I've been there since quarter to seven. No one's been in and put a line in. No anaesthetist has come and seen me. So, I've rung the missus up, I've gone, they aren't doing it today. He's having me over. This is all about earning money because everything's done for insurance. I don't like this geezer anyway. He's really rude. He's really arrogant, no one can stand him in the hospital. Horrible man. And two o', clock, three o', clock, four o', clock, this bird comes in with a tray of food. Only your token slice of dry bread, one white, one brown, one slice of cheese, one slice of ham and a yogurt. Only sometimes you got ham. Other times it was Spam or whatever. But that was another source of laughter for me, posting them on Facebook and social media. But silly little things keep me going.

So, she comes in, I said, no, I'm not allowed to eat, so I'm going down for surgery. She said, well, they told me that you can eat. I asked who told her and quickly said I'm not having a go at you, but they've told you that I can eat, but they haven't had the decency to come in and tell me I can eat. I said, do me a favour, go back to them nurses at reception and get them to get that professor up here now.

I'm sitting there, I'm absolutely fucking raging. Bear in mind, I don't like the prick, He comes strolling in with his silly goatee, beard, big old lump. Oh, yes, Mr Bates, we're not doing it today. I said, well, I've gathered that. and he looks at me as if to say, who are you answering back? I said, when did you know, you weren't going to do it? He went, a few hours ago. I said, why don't you get someone up here to fucking tell me?

He started the billy big bollocks talk about being the boss. I'm the professor. I only have to work eight hours a day. But I work from seven o' clock in the morning. I'm still here talking to you at half past six. I said, well, that's why you're the fucking boss. I said, that's why you're the professor, because you do them hours. I said, that's why you get the dough.

I stood up and he did look unnerved by my aggression, I'll tell you what, I'll go home, leave it.

He said, no, no, I'll do it in the morning. I said, I don't want you coming anywhere near me, mate. you've done one surgery with all these clips. You've rung me up and told me it isn't working. You've got me in again, right? I don't like you; I don't like your attitude. I'm going home. Leave it. So, we end the night there. I go home, everything's sorted and I'm just. I slip into a very,

very, very bad place. And the next morning I'm indoors, my wife runs Henry to school and my local doctor rings me and says, come in, I want to see you now.

So, I jump in the car and go in to see him. My wife gets home, right? Now, bear in mind, she's knowing me very well and you can see in my eyes if ok, I've always got a sarcastic little comment. I've got a quick sense of humour. My eyes smile if I've got a straight face. If you know me, you look in my eyes, you know I'm taking the piss. It's a joke. She could see the darkness that, that come over me.

This is one too many now, one too many surgeries that had been cancelled and she could see the hurt in me. She really honestly thought that I Took a drive to the Eder dam. She was beside herself. So, she rang me up, I looked at the phone, I said to my doctor, it's Bianca. I've got to answer. She went, where are you? I said, I've just come in to see my doctor. So, she said, why couldn't you tell me? I said, because he just rung me and said, come in. I'm not got washed or anything.

Bee was in tears and when I got home, she said to me, I thought you had gone to do something. And she had never felt that before. She thought it was one too many,

So, I spent the next week or so trying to get my head around the disappointment, the feeling like people were just doing now doing surgeries to have a little try at something, you would put some clips on his prostate, pull that apart, give it a wider tube. Ah, no, that's, that's not that good. We'd do an Aqua blast.

My doctor, being as great as he is knowing many great doctors because of the level he's at within the North Ryan Westphalia Medical Service, he knows a good urologist in Gelsenkirchen, which is a good two hours journey from me.

So, I go and see this, this doctor who is a fantastic man.

He reassures me that I don't need anything taken off of the prostate. So, there you go. I was going to have another operation that was going to take some of the prostate away and possibly leave me leaking everywhere and this other surgeon said there's nothing wrong with it, He X rayed to see how many clips there were, made sure they were right. he was very, very reassuring. He made sure that I was self-catheterizing properly and made sure that I had the right catheters, he gave me the right prescription for the right catheters.

I come away from there just feeling like finally I've met a doctor that don't want to chop me up or go inside and do stuff.

We're now getting to the stage where I can park up and forget the bladder's and prostate's not good, but I can live with it but I'm still having these really bad, real bad moments.

Real deep depressions and sad beyond belief.

I'm now in a position where I've decided that this probe and pacemaker in my back is not working. The doctors have agreed it's not working. And the final option was an ostomy, which is pulling your colon out of your stomach, cutting a hole in it, sewing it around, and you then live your life forever with a colostomy bag as most people know it. So, these are stick on bags that your poo comes out of. You've got no real control of it. They can be a bit windy at times. So, you know, you've now got this more mental turmoil of learning a new way to live. As if I hadn't had enough, you know. So, you know, the only things that aren't packed up down below are the kidneys, the livers, the pancreas at this stage but they're probably coming later.

I have my colostomy bag done. I wake up, I've got this new bag stuck to my belly. I can't be near people when they've had colostomies done and everything else. I'm in my posh little room on the corner looking out the window. I can see Herman the German's monument in the distance. Got me music on, I'm all right, but I've still got to come to terms with this bag. Now I joined a Facebook group before I had the surgery done and to me Facebook groups. And this is what I will say to anyone who's got a disease, concerns whether it's depression, whether it's cancer. You know, there's a group out there for everyone and you are pretty much talking to experts because they've had these things done to them. And you're also talking to people that have gone through hell and back and they're strangers, they're not judging you.

They've been through it; they've been through everything. You know, I now know some people that have, were almost dead on the table. Colon cancer, tumours, colitis, Crohn's, these people were on death's door and they have had their bags come out the other side of it. Some people six months in are still scared to go out. I'm five weeks as I write this and I'm going out. I want to go to London next Week. I want to see me boy. I want to see some pals. I've got to pluck up the courage to do things. And I've had a couple of little instances in the last five weeks where a seal's gone, but I know that you can't rush a bag change in order to get the glue right. I'm learning, but I'm doing all right but before this, what you've also got to remember with the Facebook groups is some people, when they get a health problem, it becomes their life, it defines them.

It's all they want to talk about. And some of you that know me from Facebook probably think that's all I want to talk about. But I'm not doing it for attention. I'm doing it because I don't talk to people. I put things on Facebook, it's my release. I don't talk to people and I don't ring them and ask for advice because I just don't. So, I use Facebook as my outlet. But you do get some people that a year after their stoma, they won't go out yet. They. It makes farty noises, it does this, it does that. It's basically every single thing that's bad about the stoma they will talk about and not how it's saved their lives and then you get the one, it's ones who saved their lives. They've had a couple of little farty noises in a restaurant and in the end, they go, look, I'm alive. I'm sitting in a restaurant, I'm eating dinner. I could never do that before.

So, that's the route I'm taking with this. I'm not up for any more surgeries unless it's to save my life.

I am not past all stages of depression, because it’s like being an alcoholic or drug dependent, a small thing can get you and you then allow yourself to spiral into a depression because of lack of control or fight at any given time.

Physical pain can cause this to happen to me.

I never know how I will feel in the morning, is the pain going to be so intense that I have to fight it all day, then add that to a constant voice that ants your head to allow you to sink into a negative mind set.

What I will say is that I don’t suffer massive bouts of major depression, I fight my anger issues, I am thankful for what I have as opposed to why the hell as this happened to me and the poor old Alan syndrome.

I constantly get told that I’m an inspiration or warrior and sometimes just a tough old bastard and when I used to hear this, I was embarrassed and always said that it’s the new normal and normal and I have no choice, but the truth is, you do have to be strong and take on the warrior mentality to survive this.

I don't think I am going to be able to work again physically but we don't know. I've got forty odd years of experience in construction and there must be something I can do.

I'm a member of the chartered Institute of Builders (MCIOB), along with being a member of the Institute of Engineering and Technology (MIET), they're quite big achievements for a kid from the Archway that come out of school with fuck all.

There must be something I can offer as far as works concerned but, in the meantime, my goal is out there to help others and I've got a few lived experiences, as you've read.

I am sitting here with bent toes, spasticity in my legs, medicated to the hilt just to fight of the daily pain, I use a crutch and leg brace, officially 90% disabled as assessed by the German health authority.

I piss through a tube and wear a black bag on my belly to shit in, then to top it all, I played in the snow with Henry and got a hernia, so I have a lump on my belly the size of a baby's head with a black back stuck to it, it looks like a baby's head with John Travoltas wig on it.

Chapter 27: Harry Helped Saved Me

My son Luc and his best friend took me off to the Top Gear racetrack where you can drive a Lamborghini or a Ferrari and all those flash dream cars.

Luc bought me that for my birthday. I picked up Lucs friend Harry because he lived nearer than where my son was living at the time, Harry and I were in the car and Harry's a lovely boy, albeit sends me mad at times and he's almost like having another son when you're out with them.

We went to the Euros in the summer, all the games were in Germany, and it's like having the son that you love but you've got to look out for him because he can get up to anything when he's had a drink, he's a good boy but what happened was during this car journey, we were chatting and he opened up and almost had me in tears.

This was before I was ever ill.

This was a few years ago and his dad committed suicide when he was two or three.

Harry has been tortured all these years because of his dad decision to end his own life.

He had questions like, if my dad never got my mum pregnant, he'd still be alive.

So, if I wasn't here, my dad would still be alive or my dad didn't love me enough to want to stay around, so it was my fault. He's lived with that all his life and it was heartbreaking to listen to, but I got so wrapped up in the poor me in recent years that I had never given this conversation a second thought in recent years while planning my exit from life.

Harry came over to Germany with Luc and as soon as I set eyes on him with Luc, I though what would my death do to him? What,

what would that do to Luc who's now twenty-nine, and my little boy who's coming up to seven What, what would it do to Henry, at six years old, who adores his dad?

That's what made me decide to start fighting harder. the Lokomat walking machine and things like that.

It wasn't like a rocky story but I had the choice of giving up, I was lying in bed probably eighteen hours a day and I was sharp in my answers when I spoke to my wife, I wasn't a pleasant person to be around.

She was being punished quite severely as well, in more ways than one, she's got someone, she loves but is seeing him in pain, in agony, then he's talking to her like she's a bit of shit because he's an angry man.

This is what pulled me out of it.

I started to do what was needed to get through the day and this is what I will say to people that get sad is you've got to look for little bits of little bits of happiness in everything.

No matter how sad you get, there's always something that you like.

The point of this book is for you to know my whole story and this the bit where you can snigger but I tried to simplify every thought process, albeit it is exhausting.

The energy that I was not putting to positive thinking was the exact same amount of energy that I was using up for the negative thinking, so I started switching it up.

I am not in any way going to tell you what you should do, I am however qualified enough to tell you what I did and continue to do and as I am typing this, I need a pee and that involves dragging myself to the toilet to stick a tube into my penis while having had two coffees in the hope that I can pass some output

(output is the posh word for poo) into my bag so that I can get showered and freshen up.

If anyone has been through it, **I believe that I have.**

I have visited the Eder Dam on several occasions and often look at my favourite bridge, but as part of my own self-imposed therapy, I stand there and tell myself that I have beaten you.

Back to what I do.

I had to become self-aware, critical of myself but not in a negative way but as a checking mechanism, for instance: Oi you, you prick, did you just see Bianca, Luc or Henrys face when you spoke to them.

Indicator number 1, the dark cloud is coming, I am letting it in and taking it out on people I love and who love me, even my beloved dogs would annoy me, for wanting a cuddle.

This was when I took myself away and you may find this a silly thing but if its good enough for people having panic attacks then it good enough for me.

I would regulate my breathing, not necessarily into a bag but if that gives you control then do deep breaths while constantly telling myself that yesterday has gone and I can't change it, this is my new life so don't fight it and don't worry about tomorrow, it not here yet.

I would drive to the forest and carry out this relaxing process until it passes, if it doesn't pass, I would take a nap, the problem that I find with napping on negative thoughts, you tend to wake up with the same thoughts, but I carried on the positive mantra though process while trying to sleep.

Re direction of energy:

You wake up and say to yourself, what a beautiful sunny morning, but it will probably piss with rain later.

Check yourself on the it will probably piss down with rain later, that's the negative, manage your day in bite size chunks, thinking too far ahead with a negative mind makes space for the bad thoughts to find a way in.

You can't change the fact it might rain so fuck it, grab a jacket, don't use it as an excuse to moan.

A nice passage that I have adopted that I have had printed on the back of my If it can happen to me hoodies is:

Life isn't about waiting for the storm to pass.

It`s about learning to dance in the rain.

Vivien Greene.

A big thing for me is keeping my brain active, there must be things that you enjoy, even though I can't do many things that I once loved anymore, I don't let it destroy me.

For instance, I received a post on Facebook saying that there was a motorbike show in December and it involved the European biker build off.

I know that I can't ride a Harley anymore, so instead of saying I can't have one so fuck it, I'm not going.

I put it in my calendar and planned to go on the Saturday, but sadly my body let me down, and could not get out of bed until 12pm, so Bee and I watched some Christmas films with the fire on while Henry was at his nan & grandads.

I pulled myself together and went on the Sunday, I had ice cream, took loads of photos and admired these works of art.

I had a lovely day.

Bee and I will book weekends aways or holidays, this gives me a countdown, it keeps my head straight.

By having things to look forward to, it keeps the demons at bay.

These are distractions of course and not very useful if you are not dealing with your truth and dealing with your issues, but if used in conjunction, its useful tool.

Being positive in a negative situation is not being stupid of silly, it's about survival.

None of what I am saying is easy, its hard work and takes energy, but as I say positive or negative energy are the same amount of thought process.

Being positive really helps you get through some bad times and it's also contagious, the small wins you have against the negative demons, the stronger you become.

We need to remember that a high percentage of the anxieties that you have and carry around daily, are never going to happen, what you can deal with, do not ignore it.

People tend to stress over tiny things to avoid the real issues, this leaves constant stress in that nasty compartment that is kicking at the door to make an appearance inside your head.

To make sure that this stress in your head does not affect your body with regards to exhaustion, aches and pains etc, start a journal, write your feelings down and go back to them every few days and I guarantee that you will wonder why you even stressed over them.

There is a saying that **if all the people in the world put their problems in a great big pile, and you see what others are dealing with, you would pick yours up and scarper.**

It`s about learning how to deal with our problems.

You have to live in your own head every single day and that's what being a man is all about, is not asking yourself why shit happens and dwelling on it, it's about turning up and accepting that yesterday can't be changed and putting effort into being sad about something from yesterday has to be turned around and used as a strength, such as, ''Oh well, I learned a valuable lesson yesterday'' then deal with it and move on.

Use what energy you have to defeat the negative and make it positive, nothing is easy but you must defeat the demons.

Use Facebook groups to talk to other sufferers who will support you.

Only yesterday I read in my Stoma group that a person felt alone and had no friends and having a bag stuck to her belly has ruined her life.

A simple reply from a member was that: You have 18.372 friends; we are all here for you.

What a great response.

To end this section, I will mention what I once heard.

Suicide is a permanent solution to a temporary situation.

Suicide is a way of solving or ending your problems by handing them to the people who love you.

They will carry it for life.

Human beings have been on the planet for approximately 300.000 years and during this time there has been famine, the black death, cholera, typhus and influenza plus countless wars and disputes, Middle Ages male life expectancy of 31 years old without the numbers that die at birth or infant mortality. and as a typical example of life lost is that between 1914 and 1945 an estimated 135 million people died, yet you are still here.

Your line was never broken, from the start of humanity, someone survived and reproduced to create you.

You are a miracle.

Fight against ending your **LIFE. STAY ALIVE, YOUR WORTH IT.**

PART THREE

Chapter 28: Introduction to the Stories of Strength

In this section, you will hear voices that echo resilience, courage, and transformation. These are the stories of men who have walked through fire — men who faced crippling conditions, battled the grip of alcoholism, endured illness, and carried the weight of trauma.

Each story is a testament to the human spirit's ability to rise from the darkest valleys and find light again. They remind us that strength is not about avoiding pain, but about refusing to surrender when life feels impossible.

To the men who have shared their journeys here: **thank you**. Thank you for your honesty, your vulnerability, and your willingness to turn your struggles into hope for others. Your words will inspire countless readers to believe that no matter how broken life feels, healing and growth are possible.

These pages are not just stories—they are lifelines. They are proof that even in the face of despair, there is always a way forward.

These notes are from interview recordings, so please forgive any mistakes that may occur but I thought that it was essential that we keep Jason and James's words exactly how they said them.

Overcoming Adversity: A Journey from Paralysis to Personal Growth and Public Speaking.

www.Ankerandmarsh.co.uk

JASON ANKER M.B.E (Member of the order of the British Empire for services for outstanding achievements)

Alan

Hello Jason, first off, thank you very much for taking part in the interview and openly speaking about that changed your life.

I have just noticed the football sort in the background with the words JASON ANKER MBE.

Jason

I'm a big Nottingham Forest fan.

The presented to me on the day Stuart Pierce got sacked, that's the day it was. Everyone signed it apart from Stuart Pierce, obviously. He got sacked and probably had the hump so signing the shirt wasn't high on his list of things to do.

Alan

I would like to start with asking you to introduce yourself starting with your early life prior What would we call it? The event? I suppose that I should call it what it was, the accident and then you take it from there, really. I haven't got a list of questions I really appreciate you doing this and just want to give you the opportunity to tell us your story.

Jason

So basically, not much, really. A very typical life, really.

Brought up my mum and stepdad, I lived in a pub in my teenage Years which was nice, you know what I mean.

I was in an on/off relationship with a girl from the local village that escalated. She got herself pregnant and then we ended up getting married. The usual thing happened.

Twenty-two years old I'm married, baby was born, that was in the May and in Christmas of that year I'm doing odd jobs. I've been a songwriter from leaving school. I loved it and I'm very arty. I've been made redundant at the end of 1992. So that year was basically my son's being born. I've got no job. I was a young man and picking up anything I could.

I would get work away from home on power stations, doing hard manual job, sometimes earning loads of money. But I hated it. That Christmas of 1992 I'm working with my father-in-law who ran a small roofing company, there was no real job there. It was basically giving me a job to give me a bit of cash money. A cash job to help look after us.

I had a real crap Christmas that year. Marriages failing, young marriage not getting on no money. You know I even sold my ticket in 1991, the FA cup final ticket because we had no money. That's how bad it was. So, all my life was based around football. She wasn't into football and we were just arguing constantly. It was like the final nail in the coffin. When I sold my final ticket, I found my way to get to the semi-final against West Ham. Borrowed money and then it came to it and all the coaches going down for a weekend. I couldn't afford it and weren't going to be able to justify it. So, I sold my ticket.

I 1992 it was just a bad relationship wise, wasn't getting on, splitting up, getting back together, blah blah blah. Then on the 3rd of January 1993, which was the first day back after six and a half days off and after a party the night before.

I got to work next day still drunk and not over the night before, I didn't get to bed till gone three in the morning, being picked up at seven o' clock in the morning still drunk and hungover traveling to a construction site.

All I could really do was just get through the day. Not really doing much, just toilet breaks, wandering around sites, all that sort of stuff and then as we're packing up last job of the day and again, I am thinking about Forest's and the party the night before, Forest was playing the FA cup third round on Sunday against Southampton at Forest. So, the Conversation with the four one Mates was where were we meeting what was in football what was going after football blah blah blah. So, I arrived at work a day in a low mood anyway everything's going wrong in my life and all

I'm thinking about is football and basically in my mind was get the job finished it was on TV that's why I met on Sunday get finished, get down the pub and I will catch the second half.

A job came in last minute to go and check another building where we'd not been working Went across from my father in law he goes onto a roof I follow him up there small job can't remember what job was a leak something that I can't even remember doing it to be fair I come or coming off the roof I'm first one down get to the bottom rung but at the top we had bucket of tools I'll say some there were some reasons or other for me going back up the ladder but I got about halfway and I slept and that was it, I was On the floor.

Alan

How big a fall was it, Jay?

Jason

Ten feet.

Alan

Only ten feet?

Jason

Ten feet? Yeah, just inexperienced, if I stayed with the ladder, I probably might have broken arm or something like that but I didn't instinctively jump.

There's no romantic memory of the fall it was not falling through the air or slow motion, within in seconds I'm on the floor very windy I couldn't hardly breathe so I just started winding myself I cut the back my head I felt a bit of blood so I'm rubbing the back of my head and there was this no stabbing pain around the middle, it was actually just numbness I couldn't feel my legs.

It Took about half an hour for ambulance to arrive so its Sunday no mobile phones middle of nowhere trying to get an ambulance to come they couldn't move me because I'm suspected spinal injury so they were very reluctant to even move me. I was getting really cold so decision was made to get me into the ambulance and transfer into a paramedic ambulance on the way to hospital.

Initially after an X ray I was told they couldn't find anything wrong; they were suggesting a condition known as spinal shock.

When you've had a backbone injury. You your body goes into shock and I was basically told I've been very lucky it might take a few hours, days or even a few weeks and everything be okay.

Then to be sure, the doctor sent me for a CT scan for a close look.

I obviously I knew I was going to be fine because it always happens to other people.

I was even contemplating. I always remember. It's ironic, it still stays in my mind. I gone to work that day in my favourite hoodie because I was going down the pub after work. I actually gone in my favourite ADIDAS hoodie and they cut it off of me, I was fuming. It's bizarre, isn't it? The thing that bothered me more in that moment is they cut my hoodie to get my hoodie off. Yeah, I kept saying, but it's my best hoodie. Anyway, He came back in the room. It was just the way he walked in, you know, he wasn't smiling anymore. You could tell by his face. And he didn't have to tell me. I just knew in that moment that it was bad. And he just said, yeah, you've suffered massive spinal injuries.

He said, we've had a small fracture. not a break. It hadn't broken my back. It was a small fracture. That's why it was not picked it up and again, you're thinking, well, that's good news. Well, then he said, you suffered massive spinal injuries and you'll never walk again.

That was it. It's that cold, that cold. In hindsight, I just know now you can't get involved. I understand now why they do it. If they got involved with every single patient.

They detach themselves from it completely and you understand it, more so as you get older and, you know, you go through things that must be traumatic to deal with. They'll tell someone that news but it must be traumatic for them. So, they probably desensitize from that conversation.

I understand that, but I'm twenty-four years old, I just lay there thinking, what? I was going to be all right half an hour ago.

I had some surgery next day, they put two steel rods in my back and then packed me off to a spinal unit in Sheffield, Spinal Rehabilitation Centre.

The accident happened on the Sunday, and on Friday I'm in Sheffield. It was winter, it was really bad weather. And the hospital was in the middle of nowhere on the outskirts of Sheffield, on the moors.

You go in and its people are waiting because every Friday, that's when the new patients arrive, like the intake day. Yeah, I was on bed rest for about a month, brace fitted, you are on bed rest three or four weeks, then slowly get up.

I'm not one of these people who Remember things like black and white, I don't remember days passing by and all things like that. But I knew my marriage had problems before my accident so I was convinced that was it. There's no way this was going to survive this. Yeah, but she was coming to the hospital at the time. Regular visits, you know, every day to start off with. But it was such a bad journey, you know, it was at least fifty miles away from where I lived. A real bad journey for people to come every day. And then as you go through your rehab, you're doing stuff all day long anyway.

Then at night time. that's when I started drinking with other patients. You know it was a bit weird that overnight just got drunk.

It was Just the room. You had a few beers and that. We were getting blind drunk but you were drinking every day.

I was very, not very sociable to be fair. I found it really weird that all these people would sit around in the, in the, in the recreational room rehabilitation like, like the restroom type place. Yeah, just drink and I became very withdrawn, thinking well I've not really got anything to laugh about if you know what I mean.

I made friends with a guy called David who broke his neck. He's, my age. He'd gone on a last-minute holiday with his brother. Dived into a swimming pool and broke his neck. So, he was Triplegic. He couldn't even breathe himself.

I would sit beside his bed. I would hold his drink for him and he'd have a drink and have a chat because he was into an artist as well.

He was doing a brush painting with his mouth. So, I was an artist. So, we got on every way through that but in a weird sort of way you just made me feel better. I can't imagine it would be like that. So, in a way he'd give me therapy like you know, doing anything. Thinking well at least I can do this when I leave the hospital.

January should be marked and labelled. I've been there four months, sixteen, seventeen weeks and my wife left the day that I got out of hospital. She went out on Friday night. I went out with Friends. She came back Saturday morning, so that was it, she gone.

So, I lost my wife, my legs, dignity, all them sort of things. And you're married, you have kids, so I was absolute rock bottom, but blokes being blokes, not talking about it. I just got drunk every night. Used to get blind drunk, all the problems.

I fell out of my wheelchair and broke one of the screws in my back. So, in July, I'd gone back into hospital for another massive operation. So, things going wrong. I was sort of out of control. I was very angry, very about everything. The accident, wife leaving, just everything. Like I was a victim. I didn't consciously play on it, but I was making the most of it, you know, every time I went out, there was always a group of people having affairs with mates, girlfriends and all sorts of things going, but I literally didn't care what I did. Yeah. It was like this happened to me. I don't care about anyone else. The only person I care about is myself.

My daughter starts to come to stay with for a couple of nights a week.

I would pick her up on a Monday, she stays and go back home Wednesday or Thursday. But it just made my drinking even worse. So, I wouldn't dream of it when she was there but as soon as she went home the drinking started even more so. I was drinking every day. I was taking antidepressants willingly, like, not like. It's not like today, is it? Like, you used to give me massive bottles, like one hundred tablets, so I was abusing those as well. Start taking ecstasy, start taking speed.

I couldn't do cannabis. I've never smoked, so it was like one of the drugs and I rarely did, but started getting in to the rave scene, being accepted, being in your wheelchair wasn't too bad. It seemed to be like, if anything, they may do like a beeline for you.

So, the next sort of two years just sort of passed by in a blur, really. It was literally daughter. Monday to Thursday, drink drugs Thursday to Sunday until She came to me full time mid 1994

People sort of knew what I was doing but never confronted me, it's like a known unknown, you know what I mean? So, people knew but didn't want to question it.

I was all day drinking and Some people were going to raves in Sheffield, Jay, are you coming, there's a bus, blah, blah, blah. I said, okay, then all last minute, so as you do. The pills weren't sourced from the usual source. It was a source from somebody else. A little bit cheaper than normal as well, So I was dehydrated. I've been drinking night all day, get on the coach, go to Sheffield. Took one of these tablets and I had three that night to take and took the first one. And within half an hour I was hallucinating. I was. I was all over the place. because the pills were bad, a lot of people were struggling a little bit as well, but nothing like me.

So, we eventually got back onto a coach. At this point, I'm hallucinating, I am thinking that everyone's trying to attack me. It was just awful. Got on a bus, drove fifty miles back to Newark. My friends all panicking, not knowing what to do. Just dropped me in the hospital and left me. All right. So, my dad got a call like three in the morning, your sons in the hospital. We think he's dying. So, mum and dad rushed to the hospital. I'd had a massive allergic reaction to all the stuff I'd taken, I Got rushed through Queen's Medical in Nottingham. Put in an induced coma. And that's where I stayed for seventeen days, basically fighting for my life. Wow.

Dad would be advised to turn the machine off. At one stage. He was told that I've got brain damage and there was nothing that the hospital could do, but after seventeen days, I actually woke up.

The biggest issue was that had been through hell and had tracheotomy and the doctor couldn't get it out, as soon as he went to do it, the blood pressure on the sides went through the roof. He thought it was going to give me a heart attack.

So, no one would actually take it out and by chance another member of staff was there and he wasn't even a doctor, he just came in and just took it out straight away in one sort of motion. He got it out. But with a fight, I couldn't speak, obviously. You got a hole in your throat, you can't speak. I'm hallucinating Even though I was conscious, I was just hallucinating all the time. It's like just horrendous things happen in the hospital. I thought it was trying harvest my organs. Crazy stuff that going through your psych, you know, psychological reckoning of what was happening was really, really bad. That played out for a couple of weeks. Didn't recognize the kids. They come Draw me pictures. It wasn't them. They put pictures of my kids. It was. I knew it wasn't them even though it was them, I was like really hallucinating really bad.

It was very similar to having a stroke.

I had done even more damage. I couldn't. I couldn't move my arms properly. Couldn't speak even when. When they tracked it up, blah blah, blah. Couldn't get many words out. I was repeating myself. Everything was like massive ball of confusion.

I Spent nearly five months in hospital. They ended up shoving me in a stroke unit.

They didn't know what to do with me so the Doctors ended up moving me in to a stroke unit. It was basically learning to feed myself. Speak again. I could speak but you were like speak properly. Which I still suffer with speech today. My slurring all come from the drugs.

The effect of brain damage left me speech impediment.

When I was released from hospital people were different towards me, the Sympathy everywhere had gone.

When I came out, people's attitude was like, well he didn't have to do drugs.

It was my problem and self-inflicted. Mum was fine. But other people around in the village was a bit like well he is just a druggie? So, you'd lost a lot of that sympathy.

Then pressures hit me now, you know, from parents like don't do anything like that ever again. So, from that moment I decided that I'm going to pretend to be okay, and that would stop people who cared about me from worrying so much, even though inside, I was a proper angry man.

So that's where many of my problems stemmed from, I think I've always suffered anxiety anyway. But that's when I first realized I was struggling. But I caused so much pain to everybody else. The guilt that I felt was I can't put people through this no more.

I Was told I couldn't drink anymore because of brain damage; I still like to drink but it has a different effect. Sometimes I have two pints, and it'd be like I've had about ten or twenty, I'd be absolutely blind drunk. So, I was still causing a lot of problems with my friends.

It was like babysitting when I went out. So, I used to go out feel so conscious about being in a wheelchair that drink became less of my go to.

At this point I went back to counselling. And I was taught About the one to ten theories. Always try and be the opposite.

Everything's got an opposite. So, to try and think that everything's got this Opposite way. it was bizarre and extremely difficult to explain to you. But I got number five one day. And after six months of counselling, I got the number five on his scale, And the question I asked the councillor was, well, fives got no opposite. Five's just five. It's just okay. Which meant, weirdly, I learned this coping mechanism that nothing really excited me and nothing really got me down. I stayed in the middle; you have to work sometimes. I would go to a funeral and not work myself up to be as sad as I should be, equally if went to a wedding or something positive. I just bring myself down all the time.

So of course it was like I found a way to cope. So, there was weeks where Abbie would come to my house, So I stay in, but as soon as she went home, I'd go out, so Thursday night I would pretty much drink until Sunday night and then when someone was back in the week was looking after them. I'll be at school to pick em up. Do Tea one night and the following weekend, it was my weekend to go out drinking. So literally, I found a way. Every two weeks, a rota, this is my coping mechanism to get through each two-week period.

So, for a day, I found a cycle of every two weeks being the same. Same cycle. It was every two weeks and that was my life. Very luckily, I fell into disabled water-skiing scheme. I saw an advert when I had been in hospital in 1995. When I came out, it was September and SI kept seeing these adverts on the tv, local news, about disabled waterski charity, in Nottingham. it was pretty much the end of season, actually, like the last session of the year, so, like end of middle of September, I'd gone water skiing.

It's the first thing I'd done, of all the things I had tried and done after my accident. Wheelchair, tennis etc, wheelchair everything involved a wheelchair,

Well, waterskiing didn't. You are on water. You're on a special ski, here was no wheelchair. I was like hooked from the moment I did it the first time. Dragged out the water with two blokes either side, I was on an adapted ski. And it was something else I'd got to look forward to.

A couple of times a month through the summer, you go off water skiing, either in Nottingham or wherever and bizarrely, the kids started socializing with other people with disabilities.

So, you go water skiing and the people with no legs, blind, no arms. So, the kids sort of grew up around people with disabilities, so it's like becoming normal for them.

So that was really good for me.

I'm still using alcohol as my go to therapy. My counselling is finished. He signed me off. It Was a bit like I'm in a council flat, It was like mom and dad really helped out, but I'm in a council flat no prospects and I thought this is my life now I've got to make the most of it and it's sort of what I did in a way that two week cycle was there drink kids, drink kids, drink kids and that was enough, if you know what I mean?

People say would you ever suicide after your accident and for me the whole thing with depression and suicide is that. people don't start off on day one at suicide there's a journey they go down.

The majority of people they get so low it's terrible but that line of crossing to take your life is the final step. Yeah, for me there's so many people at this stage that might never take their own life but they're not far from the line, It's a line.

I'm into it it's not much more to go from I'm so pissed off being depressed. So did I have suicidal thoughts and I made reckless choices. I didn't care if I lived or died. But for me as my child my real dad wasn't there for me when I was so young that I was so angry and this made me think that I'll always be always there for my kid.

My kids were enough to make me continue to fight what each day brings and fair play to my ex-wife.

She let me have my kids so my I brought my kids up by myself, I don't know where I'd be if I hadn't had that, if I didn't have the kids to bring up, I don't know what I would have done so there was enough to spare me from ever getting that low but I thought if you haven't got me your mum's no good. So, I felt obliged to bring my kids up yeah which was good, they are what kept me going from day to day to be fair, you know going to school, dropping off at school pick up doing the tea so I just became a parent that was it so.

People say was your life gone? It wasn't great, but you know looking at other parents, fathers, working fathers I went to every school play I went to every sports day so I you know that was it for me my kids were everything and as kids are getting older know turned to teenage years and my daughter left when she was fifteen so she couldn't live with me anymore because my behaviour then becoming more noticeable.

Instead of drinking when the kids weren't there, I started drinking and they start to see the demon side of it if you know what I mean. So, she to go back to live with her mom when she was fifteen. So now Sam is going through the boy stuff and because I'm now drinking whether he's there or not as well. Not so much at home I didn't really drink. I'm not a massive home drinker but you know we go out and Sam will come along.

So, by the time the end of the night he's wheeling me home making sure I get in bed so he starts to see things he shouldn't be saying. Yea

In 2017 I got my compensation. I should have got in 2015 but the Royal Court of Justice were pissing about.

So, all of a sudden, you've got this person Who's at this time is depressed or was it more anxiety, probably both.

I just couldn't see a future. So yeah, and it was all anxiety based. All future based. What I'm going to do.

I received £408.000 so what do you do? you start spending, all of a sudden, I've got money in the bank. We put into trust. It was bizarre. It was set up put me into trust. You can still claim your benefits.

I wasn't comfortable this this situation but anyway, I'm now battling my anxieties that I've got this money but I'm claiming benefits even though it was all legal rules you have to follow. This felt so uncomfortable. So, I started spending a lot of time in Tenerife. I could all day nice hotel. I'd spends £10.0000, going over there for about a month, two months.

I'll go back to Tenerife again then spent some time about two months in Tenerife over Christmas.

I got approached by somebody who'd heard my story its hat weird how it happened.

A guy was working close to me and there's a guy Called Ian Whittingham, who was a real big speaker. He was in a wheelchair.

He was an active speaker. He was taken Poorly. It was a bizarre. One of the most bizarre conversations, where this guy who lived down our street, He wasn't a friend, id Say hello to him every day. When I saw him, he was working at this factory where this guy was supposed to be speaking and at lunchtime he was just chatting with Dan, who was the trainer. and Dan said, oh, today a guy called Ian was supposed to be here today he's in a wheelchair, but unfortunately, he's taken poorly. This guy said, I know someone in a wheelchair. That's it Wouldn't ever have happened. That's how random it was. But then I'm down the pub, I'm drunk, I get given this business card with his name on, get told his story. Do you fancy doing some speaking about your accident and when you're drunk? Oh, yeah, I can do that.

I woke up next morning and you check your pockets, look to try and figure out how much money you've spent for all your change. There's this business card and I thought I'd give the Guy a ring. I rang him up, went to meet him, told him the story. He said, yeah, his name was Dan Terry. Yeah, I think that there's a story in there, definitely and it must be told.

I went on his first job with him, sat back and I thought, well, it's not for me. I can't do that. No chance. He rang me up about a week later. What do you think? So, I said, I can't. I can't do that. It's not my bag. No, never thought of doing it like before. It's not me.

When I am not drunk, I don’t really say a word to anybody.

He left me and then he rang me out of the blue a couple months later. I'm going to take you somewhere else. Come out with me again. I'll take it to a different place. Just to get another view of the process, So I went and watched him and then right at the end of the session, he said, oh, Jason, he's got a couple of words to say, which I hadn't. So, he really put me on the spot. So,

I just rambled through my story, and at the end one of the people in the room says, that was really impactful.

Knowing Dan like a do, that was a plan. He told the guy to stand up and me that without a doubt. I know now that's the encouragement I needed. Yeah. You know what I mean? And then from there it just sort of grew. I thought, yeah, I'm going to do this, I suppose I'm going to have to show him a story.

Dan is sadly not with us anymore, RIP.

I used to swear a lot. I so nervous. Bright red on stage, enjoy doing it. But I can remember always speaking. It's probably this story I tell. It's probably not exactly how it happened, but over years it changes around a bit, but on one occasion a guy was sat in the room at the front of the presentation, looking everywhere, twitching, looking down, not listening.

I used to be very different from now. I didn't tell people anything about some really personal bits, I only told the bits that I think you want to know. So, I just came out with it. To get his attention I said ``Can you imagine being incontinent? Can you imagine wearing a leg bag`` I just. I just let rip. I don't know where it all came from. It just all came out. Once it started, it never stopped. But at the end of the session, he made a point of coming to shake my hand. He said I get it now. So, it's like in that moment I also I got it.

So, if I share my story, it's just a story but one person did something different and that young man coming to shake my hand changed things. That was the only emphasis I needed. And my attitude was now, I'm going to do this.

Working with Dan, who used to run a day long BAL behavioural safety course, I would sit there, do my fifteen minutes, start of the day, then just sit in the audit, sit in the crowd, just listen to Dan talk about all behavioural safety stuff. So over that eight months to a year when I was working with Dan, I picked up so much knowledge about safety. You start using the correct terminology and phrases.

I was down to do a job by myself in Scotland. We're still working with somebody else, a guy called Matt Terry. Not related, but Matt and Dan used to work together. Not related family wise, but the same surname. Matt was doing a joint job in Scotland, Aberdeen for Robert McAlpine’s. So, a big job. I got a presentation on a computer and on the day, I was traveling up to Scotland, Matt rang me, said, I can't make it. I had an accident, an accident on his motorbike or something. I can't make it. So, I'm there thinking I've got to go on my own.

I'm on a train with a computer, I actually had a little bit of a presentation to do and it went down really well. So, it was a bit like, well, I could do this by myself. I don't have to be with other people.

I don’t need a security blanket and it went from there.

I think what people like was that I turn up in My jeans. Because that is what I was my comfortable in, I couldn't be anyone else wearing suits and being different, I could only do it the way I wanted to do it.

My first big job was working for Babcock’s. they said they wanted me to speak at their main conference.

Their director said No one can use him before he speaks at the main conference.

We have some problems down the shipyard down in Devon. I need him down here. I just need him down here now because the project has got massive problems. So, I took myself out, and off down to Devon. Sat in the foyer of the officers and then met Andy Forbes,

He said, the moment I saw you, I knew he was going to be perfect. Your stood there in your trainers, your jeans, your hoodie.

This is the type of person I need to tell a story. So that's how it was.

I always aimed every word at the operatives, always aimed at the worker at the coal face.

My presentation was a story like, don't be like me, do not be like me. I'll tell you this horrible story, but don't be like me and I suppose back then in the late in 2009/2010/2011 & 2012 that's what safety wanted. DON'T BE LIKE ME

As you know, I started getting a really good reputation. It was mainly on construction. It was mainly porta cabins. Speak to lads off site and there's always issues with people walking out of the meeting rooms, concrete just going. and I was really busy, basically on-site chaos.

I was working four or five days a week, every week and earning decent money. It's like. It was weird. But it's like the money didn't mean anything to me. I'd spend it as soon as it came in. I was buying all sorts of cars. It was a brand-new Audi on the drive and all these things, The illusion that you're doing okay. Yeah, that illusion but really, I'm struggling, but people are going to see this other side of me.

When I was drunk, Jason's always in a good mood. Jasons all right, the wheelchair drunk, making lot of People laugh.

So, this Persona I created was, was, was that the only person I could never hood wink was my mum because she would say, what's up with you? I said I'm fine mum. I used to tell her. She always says you're not but I always say mums always know. You can't hide anything from your mom.

By now business started really picking up. Abbie came to work for me.

I couldn't keep up with book work. I was trying to do the books invoices, trying it all myself. I'm working weekends all spent doing paperwork. I thought this is ridiculous.

So, Abbie came to join me. She was working at a bank and trying to do my book work, invoices, getting the hotel sorted out. Then things started really taking off and I talked her into leaving the bank completely going work to be full time. Which she did

Sam stopped going out with me, listening to my story every day and to be fair, looking back now, it was probably the right thing for him to do because he was having to listen to all the bad stuff every day.

So, he left. He didn't stay long, stayed about six months. He aids I can't do this so he left.

Business wise and outwardly I'm really starting to succeed. business picking up. Yeah, I get all the speakers on board an agency started to form. So outwardly I'm doing really well, really really well financially I'm doing well. Money in the bank booked up for like a year in advance, So I would look at my diary and I'm full for a year so I suppose I wasn't flash and bragging but I could go and play cards and lose two hundred quid, you know, and didn't matter. I would take it down lose basically.

I would say I was fashionable but it didn't mean anything to me. I seemed to have loads of money but it wasn't the answer for me. Yeah. You know, and people around said he must be all right now, look, he's got a nice house, got cars. So, you've lost it a little bit, you've lost that support because people think oh, he's all right now. Yeah, especially when you went out and the conversation. Was well you're compensated now. Your life should be all right.

I'm doing really well financially but Relationship wise, it's just disaster. If I'm drunk, I'll chat anybody open, blah, blah, blah, but when sober I realized I was going to live in a wheelchair.

I've moved to a nice little bungalow. Brand new bungalow. Yeah. Say brand new, but off nephew live there for about six months. I've got a lovely bungalow, nice car drive, money in the bank, but I was dreadfully unhappy. What's the point of all this?

It means nothing to me and then I came home from work one day and there's a letter and it's been a really stressful, hard week and there's an official letter to be honest, I thought it was a call to jury service and that is the last thing I need.

The envelope had the royal crown on it and the reason I'm pissed off is because the I subject had been mentioned by some mates, like in passing, in the weeks before. So, I was being called up. So, it literally got me. I was thinking, this is all I need. I can't. I can't do this.

As always, my head ran away with itself and I finally I read it like, and I've been nominated for an MBE a Member of the British Empire for outstanding achievements.

So, I read it, I thought, oh, wow. So that's amazing. So, you're not to be nominated, like, then had a cup of tea, sat down, ready property, and now you've got it.

I have actually been awarded an MBE. Wow. But you can't tell anybody at that moment.

This is probably about November time, and the reason that you are not allowed to tell anyone is because It's announced in the New Year's honours list.

You get such amazing news, but you can't tell nobody. It's like. So, it's like Okay.

So, I obviously told my parents when it was time as well. I told them, obviously everyone's over me walking on that. And it was. But it's bizarre that it didn't mean anything to me like it should have done because I just know I'm in such a bad place this, this. But on the day. So, we've got in New Year and it's like June time, you get down to the thing. My dad came with my daughter and like for my dad, I was absolutely made up. My dad was like, amazing. But for me it meant nothing. It just felt nothing.

Alan

That's such a shame though, isn't it? Because of all the hard work you're doing and how you're helping in People and you can't see it because at.

Jason

This point I'm very unaware about my anxiety was yeah, I've lived it for so long it was like the normal I would say to people when I finally started opening up about things.

Not one of my friends believed me, how have you suffered? They couldn't understand how. How bad I've been suffering. But then once you start explaining all these events that evolved over the years the affairs drink all them things start to make sense to people, so they missed it completely. And yet when it all came out that my whole life is built around anxiety in the future and what's going to happen, I felt in the past that's sort of gone it was all future based life with disabilities what's it going to be like when I'm older, all those things just constantly going round and round and round,

In 2015 life has started to come sort of okish over a month I was and then I was. I was quite happy as well. I was like yeah this is all right. I'm comfortably off, don't need anything. I'm all right. My drinking I wasn't binging as much so I probably about once a week I still get drunk when I was out but it wasn't like Friday, Sunday anymore it wasn't drinking really calmed down yeah busy. I found new purpose. I was traveling around a lot different hotels, different locations so I suppose I was okay. And then it was again oh you need a girlfriend. I wasn't particularly looking for one because I thought I don't know if I want that or not. I don't think that is it but maybe it is, maybe it's not. Maybe that's missing piece to the old thing and then bumped into an old school friend and we started chatting and blah blah blah. Next thing we're in a relationship and it went really really quick far too fast.

Twenty-five years and I've been relationship my girlfriends but nothing like moving in, all this it happened really fast and but people's like got caught up in the old romantic thing involved this is the icing on the cake.

Finally, it's got someone blah blah blah.

Alan

So, would you say that they wanted it more for you than you wanted it for you?

Jason

Yeah, initially without a doubt. It was like you know was always the pressure you know if only had a girlfriend now everything be hunky dory and blah Blah, blah. So anyway, it happened and it was a bit of a whirlwind and blah, blah, blah. Everything was going really well for a good, good year. Not really arguing at all. Old school girlfriend. Oh, this is probably the best it's going to get for me, you know, this is all right. She was pretty girl at school. She's still pretty. Everything was good she was divorced, got her own house, running her own business. So, I thought it's not even like a financial thing, it's just fun but it turned out business wasn't as great as what she said it was and we moved into a house together. I think it lasted two months in the house, So I live in this massive cottage in the middle of nowhere. Two acres of land that I work away from. She's left.

I've got home from working away. I've been a really hard week. And when I drove home and it was raining, I dropped my mate off at his house. Drove about ten miles away from village where I lived, ten miles away, middle of nowhere, thinking, what the hell have I done here? Middle of nowhere, this is it, what I'm going to do. And then I drove onto my driveway and I just looked at the house, looked at my driveway. I thought I live here. This is amazing. Yeah, it's massive. It's like the dream cottage I've always dreamed of. So that then became my obsession, the house. Do what I'm going to do, I'm going to renovate the house. That's what I'll do. I'll spend all my time renovating. That's what I've done for the last sort of eight, nine years is really renovated the house. But the point from that moment was I decided to search into something. So, I've looked at Buddhism, looked at all these things, self-help things, Teddy Robbins, done them all.

I've done things, one thing. So, I would look at Self-help and how my wellbeing could be affected or influenced my life. The choice I made. So, I literally just decided I was going to change my life.

It was like a choice. I'm going to start doing these things. These people tell you like you breathe a nice thing. Oh yeah, there. That never worked. I thought, you know what, I'm going to start giving these things a try. So, I started doing some breathing which really helped my anxiety. And then you do things for thirty days, couple of months and you start. I feel a little bit better. I do something else that's what I've done for the last eight years. I got the nine steps that I've done. The diet, gratitude, sleep. I get to bed at night being grateful for things. And it's amazing how things started to change and I started to realise that It's the way that you think that is the secret.

Nothing's changed. Your life is your life is your life. Yeah. Just the way you see things and think about things changes the way you look at things. I know you're into this because you, you want this. You can't change what's happened. You just change how you build it. It's all to do with your attitude. Your attitude becomes everything.

So, once I start changing my attitude, I use it on the talks to, I would say is that I used to wake up and the first thing I'd always see was a wheelchair beside my bed. So, you start off the day with that poxy wheelchair ruined my life. It's there every day no matter where I go or What I doit is there every day. Whereas what I changed my attitudes now I'm grateful every morning wakes up

I'm grateful. Wheelchair's there, if I didn't have it beside my bed, I can't do anything. The wheelchair has given me the opportunity to do things that I would never have got to do, To the places I've been, things I've seen would never have happened if I'd not have my wheelchair.

I frame it really well. I say my wheelchair has taken me further in life than I could imagine. Except look at me on stage thinking I wish I wasn't in it, but I am. The only thing I changed about wheelchairs is my attitude. Since I've done that, my life's changed completely.

I started making these steps and changed in my life. But I'm still drinking. I'm still drinking. I. I came to a conclusion. I Woke up New Year's Day about five years ago and I said I'm not drinking anymore. It wasn't a constant. I might start drinking soon. But I woke up.

Relationships weren't nice when I was drinking, everything I can go back to, I would say drink was always the Core. The main thing. Dream. It was always. It was always present. Yeah. And all my things I'd done that went wrong. Drinking was always a constant. And as always there and ultimately probably my biggest downfall.

I sort of know now. My kids went through the years of fifteen, sixteen, seventeen, eighteen and we're going to Tenerife all the time and they must have been terrified. Dads getting drunker and drunker. How was I being going to get into bed. I didn't know that they were living the anxiety of me drinking.

You know, basically. What's dads going to do tonight? Basically, just say the wrong comment and he would kick, someone said one thing to me. I was awful.

So, when I woke up, I didn't think I'd stop forever. I thought I'm going to stop for thirty days because my anxiety. I noticed my anxiety got a bit out of control again. I thought. So, I'm trying not drinking for a month. So, no pressure. Didn't really say anything to anybody. Really. I just. I stopped drinking. And then after a month, I just noticed a bit of difference in this straight away.

I was in more control. I was. I was like more in control of my thoughts and moods than they controlled me.

My anxiety is always present. I'm not going to lie. I still suffer to this day. I know it's there. But bizarrely.

I don't do as much now. This Was how I used to do it? My anxiety was Like a person that lived on my shoulder as long as I knew it was on my shoulder. It wasn't in my head.

So, things would happen. I literally glanced over my shoulder to see if it was there or not. So, it wasn't there. It was in there.

I could do. So, it was like the things I did to look after myself was to keep my anxiety on my shoulder and out of my head, it’s still there out to this day. But it's not this massive thing anymore. It's like this tiny little thing sticks us there. Yeah. And then the errors I used to do was always like past or future. So whenever, again, I don't do this anymore. But at least I used to put them there. If I felt bad, I literally put my hand there. Think of what I was thinking about. It was either I got drifted back into the past or I was worried about the future again. All I literally did was get my hand and place it and make Myself cantered again and back to the present moment. Because that's all we ever really have. We've got nothing. We haven't got. All the things you've been through have gone. You can't change that. But all things you worry about haven't even happened.

Everything in your future is a result of what you do in this moment. That's why I'm very present today. That's why my gratitude is a big part of my wellbeing. But people still think it's a thing you do then you just carry on. They don't get the well beings forever. So, what happened this year was. Which is still again part of my story. So, I talk about this journey I've been on but rebuild your life. It's. It's getting here getting to the present moment. Once you get into present moment that's when you start to control things. Because if you put all your effort into one thing which is now, you're not worried about you.

You aren't got time to worry about all these things. If everybody is not present. Then you'll drift off into the past. And also, you catch yourself thinking where he was ten years ago.

It was the same every anniversary of the accident the same.

You start end of December. I start feeling it coming. I start drinking Christmas drinking to get to the third of January. I build myself up this massive down every year I'd be angry with everything and even twenty years later when I was in Scotland. We're going away for the new year. It's the 2nd of January I'm in Edinburgh for a couple of days. I woke up in the morning twenty years I've been a wheelchair twenty years and it ruined the whole day. I couldn't shake this fever; you know twenty years ago. All you've lost going over football. The old things just came rolling back all the things I lost. And then now I always work now. I try my hardest. Even when I was working, I have January off work. I wouldn't work in January. Yeah, all the time. And I'm off where it's the most important time of the year for safe to be at work. It's January, such a bad month for accidents things now I make a point. I work every January third like oh man. It's part of the service because It's not what happened to me that cause the problems. It's just how I dealt with it. The wheelchair was never a problem. Yeah, the wheelchair was Never the problem. It was my attitude about the wheelchair was always a problem. Yeah. And the perceived things I put in my head. So, relationships were. It's not going to last.

My attitude to everyone was that I know you don't get it. So, I don't bother you about me being in a wheelchair.

I talk myself out of everything. And obviously you can allude to it because that's what you do. You talk to yourself Alan, don't you? Yeah. He's got a wheelchair. Can't do this in a wheelchair. Can't have kids. But all the time I pushed so many people away. Yeah. Who probably would have made really good life partners. I pushed them all away.

I convinced myself that it'd be a matter of time before you leave. So, there's no point starting, just push people away.

So, this year it's happened this year as well. But I'm more conscious than last year. It's the same. I probably work till the second week in December. That's always been with cut off. I mean. But last year some work got moved and I broke up. Which I actually break up on Monday. Those work in January this year. So, I broke up really early in December. And all of December off and all of January off. Like two months off work. I'm not working, so some of the things to do for wellbeing are things to do for myself. All things I do. I've had to invest the money. So, all of last year I got myself a speech therapist.

I know I talk slow slightly still. Especially when I get loose talking. But I can go on stage now. Especially on stage. I can really form my words properly. So, I had two lessons a week. Went down to two a month, then one a month. And towards the end I think I'm okay now. So that was an investment. Having lessons. Fifty pounds a lesson.

I use Mark Wilkinson as a life coach. No matter how busy I am I make time to do two sessions a month where I paid to speak to somebody who could be about business, about personal stuff, about how I'm feeling. Just have someone. But it's a cost. It's a cost there.

So, because I don't drink anymore. That's what I spend my money on and you're investing in yourself, Which drink doesn't do.

What I say to people is the only investment, the only person you can look after is yourself.

Is that That's selfish. No, it's selfless. Because if I can be a better person. That radiates another people.

My relationship with daughter the best it's ever been. Now she's so relaxed that dad's not getting drunk no more, That's amazing. Sam's always suffering his mental health. Lived with me really rock relationship with Sam kicked him out. He was eighteen. Running a flat for a bit paid for that. He'd trash it just then he. When he was living with his grandparents, I gave him another job and he was just giving him money. So, he comes back to live here during lockdown. he had nowhere to live. He's going to come back. I'll pay rent and all that blah blah for a few months. Still here. Thirty-three still here. it's been rocky being here. We'd have arguments all the time. I get really get anxious with him. But on this new thing, I believe that if you want people to change, you got to change yourself.

You can't change everybody. You can't expect someone else to change. So, I started to change the relationship with Sam. He was very, very wary at the start thinking kid, so dad, you learned all these new techniques. It's not a technique. It's the way I'm living now. It's took the best part of six months for him to trust That's who I am now. because dad used to be a kick off dad but I don't do that anymore. I literally don't do it anymore. So now and then he has an issue and I say come talk to me and he knows dad will listen. Dad won't give advice, say this or won't do that. just says what can I do to help? Yeah, you tell me what I can do mate. I'll help you so well that's taught me thirty-two years of being in a wheelchair probably since I've stopped drinking, I stopped being so selfish.

I can't help anybody else to help myself. Yeah. So, before it was all like don't worry about me. I'll try helping people. Oh, so it's like now. my presentation now has changed. The presentation is don't be like me. My presentation is be like me. Because if I go back to my accident. If I had been the person I am today, I would have had my accident.

I wouldn't to be in that off mood I was in that day. Ah it. I would not be my angry person when I'd arrived on site.

A good Night's sleep. If I had marriage problems today, I would probably have told someone about the problems. Do you know what I mean? It's all about that's part of it.

So, my life now is like I've never been in a wheelchair.

I go to bed at night, how I wake in the morning, and I feel sorry for some people who have a normal life but do not seem to have a purpose.

How'd you get out of bed in the morning without a purpose? What is it that drives you out of bed? What is it? A life without purpose is unbelievable.

So, my personal purpose is to live with passion. If you're not passionate, you can't do what you have to do and I wouldn't be able to do what I do and that's why I have integrity, I'm still working on me. I've still got a Couple of things I've got locked up there. I'm still not there yet but I'm working on it.

I try to be more open to people, I'm still not the best at saying what I really think.

I'm still the old me. I don't want to upset people. I know that's a trait I've got and I've not got rid of that. I could never upset people; I'd rather me lose out.

Love is a massive one, after my accident, I hated himself. Then after the drugs, I've literally despised myself for years. So, like I said, how could I keep in a relationship and love someone when you despise yourself?

I just hated everything about me. So, I was the cause of all this and then when you realize you've had an accident and as you get older and see that it's not my fault.

When my mum passed away a couple years ago. She had nightmares with me. I was horrendous. Years and years of me turning for Christmas Day and ruining it and kick off and throw cans at the walls and I mean that until know you've ruined lives. Not just because I'm in a wheelchair, but because of the way I acted the way I was. And I'd always justify it as well. To myself yeah. Imagine you don't live in a wheelchair. Imagine my life, it was always about me you know what I mean it was like that was the go-to excuse and no matter what I did I would never say sorry because I was cursed and living in a wheelchair.

That's what it's used on people but I'm so grateful that my mum started to see the change in me when I stopped drinking.

She passed away two years ago but I stopped drinking. She sees the change in my emotions and my mum started to see the change in me which just meant everything still does. Now she's gone it means even more to me that she saw it and that the change didn't come after mum had passed, she started to see that I changed.

So now when I do my presentations there's a small element of safety in there obviously. But the biggest thing for me is when people say oh, I AM YOU. You've made me realize IM YOU. Everything you described about your life falling apart and sleeping on the sofa having no more blah blah blah. I'm you. I'm you now so we can help more people.

The Safety world I was in for so long. I don't call myself a safety speaker anymore. I try my hardest. I don't go through a long-winded accident story like most people do. I thought I'm on a building site. That's my accident story. I'll tell you what I'll tell about my life after that happened. I'm not going to go oh, it was a rainy day and the sun was shining. It's not about that. But that's what I did, but I now say that these are the consequences of what happened to me. But actually, the majority of that happened was because of my mindset of I hate the world. Acceptance is good but you need it to be total acceptance.

When you accept something, it always felt like it was a weakness.

Why should I accept your behaviour? Because you've done something wrong.

Whereas now is I don't care what your behaviour is. I'm really calm if I concentrate on myself so what happens? I can't control now is making sure that I am in total control of me.

The only time I wanted to have a drink was when I was the at end about two months when I really suffered mental health. It's was close I almost started to drink again. I've still got a cupboard in my house full of whiskey. I used to Go traveling around Scotland and buy the most expensive bottle of whiskey I could afford, but it's still there.

Never dream of touching it. You know I'll never have a drink again. I'll never drink again because it, because of all the negative things that alcohol causes and since I've stopped drinking it's like it's made looking after myself so much easier.

I could never not drink. I'm not even a preacher. I don't even say do it; I can't. I don't want to be exposed to drinking.

I tell people benefits the benefits I found for me. All I'll say is the only thing I do is try to be more be more conscious of why you're drinking. If you’ve had a really hard stressful day alcohol's probably not the best way, go to.

Alan

What's been lovely for me to listen to is the coping mechanisms that you have to learn for yourself. You can't be told them. You have to learn for yourself. And once you've learned that you need it then you can seek help for new ways of doing it. And, and there's been things that you've said that I've grinned. Not because I'm finding it funny is I've wrote all my stuff in the book now this is the last part and you've said so many things that I've had to learn in a short time. You've got the, the length of journey on me but the self-awareness, you know, the little voice on your shoulder keeps him out, don't let him in. Be aware that he's there and don't you know all of them things are the things that I'm still in the process of learning, you know. So, listening to you talk about it is just absolutely fantastic. Not because I want you to have suffered, but the idea of doing this is to not let other people suffer if they read it.

Jason

The bit that's really resonated with me was people said do you wish you'd done this sooner? And I'll say first thing is I don't even think about that because I can't change it.

What's happens for me, this was the right length of journey for me.

You change when the time is right for you.

If I'd have changed earlier, the life we live now wouldn't happen.

My story is not all the bad stuff. I couldn't go and say, so I had an accident and I'm now fine. What sort of story is that?

Yes, I had an accident. I've got my kids and I've got a big cottage over two acres of land.

So, the other issue I've always had is motivational or inspirational. A lot of these speeches on safety start out as a motivational safety speech but unfortunately, motivation doesn't last very long. People are motivated to start a diet. How long does it last? But people are motivated to get to the gym. How long for? When you're inspired to do something that is forever.

That's that inner voice also. You're doing it for yourself. You'll be inspired to do something for yourself.

There are some people I know, Sean Rose an example. So, I met Sean when I was water skiing. Sean came along, just had his accident like a year before. Got a water ski, was skiing around the lake like he'd been all his life.

It was the next army guy who broke his back snow skiing. So now Sean Rose has been a world champion water skier. He's been a world champion at the X Games snow skiing. He's now a fully certified pilot. Sean's never had a bad day. Right. He had a stillborn daughter die; He had a baby. It died for about thirteen weeks. And he's one of these people who just Never lets it get him down. And for me that's been a problem for me, not from Sean, is that most of these motivational speakers, even inspirational speakers, are people who had an accident, climbed Everest the next day.

For ten years I could hardly get out of bed, but they find everything easier, these people had these positive inspiring nothing will defeat them attitudes before their accidents. They are soldiers, They're different. They're a different animal to us, they're freaks. They are lovely, but they're freaks.

The majority of People are like me and you, Alan, we can't do that. And all they do is make me feel bad.

They sit there and these guys are going, oh, I'm in a wheelchair and I was doing this or that the other day, I feel like saying, oh well done to you, because it makes me feel like crap, because I can't do that.

In fact, one of my presentations I use a story of W. Mitchell.

I actually reached out and made contact with him.

He wrote a book called, ITS NOT WHAT HAPPENS TO YOU.

So, his story. This is what I allude to. I use his example. So, this guy Left the Marines, Navy or whatever it was, He's got on his big motorbike. Looking at all the young ladies on the sidewalk and posing and as he looks up a lorry crosses his path. So, he gets his motorbike to the slide on his side like in a Proper movie. So, he slides under the lorry and comes out the other side, like not a scratch on him. He's obviously trapped under his motorbike and as he is struggling to get away from being trapped under the bike, The petrol lid come off his off his tank. So, his petrol everywhere and it all goes up in flames. Now this guy's been burnt to a crisp. Lost his fingers, just completely burnt, nothing Left his arm still.

His Injuries are that bad, they can't give him pain relief. His injuries are that bad. He got no pain relief. The nurse can't understand why. With such pain. Every day he is saying, good morning. They're like, this guy should be thinking his life's ended, like the other patients He wasn't. So, after a long time he became a mayor, climbed a mountain, become a millionaire. He learned to fly a plane. So, he carried all this with no fingers and massive disabilities. So, to recap he became a businessman. He's Got a pilot's license; he buys a plane. So, he's got some customers on this plane going to take off and the plane crashes. Just takes off and crashes. So, the four people, that plane walk out uninjured, but he's paralyzed, he is now paralysed.

So, he's been burnt to a crisp in one accident, has another accident. Like five years later he's in a wheelchair, he's paralyzed and his wife leaves him but he refused to give up. He just believes that life is amazing. But as I said, these are the freaks. You say people are like that, you know what I mean? So, it's, it's like, how do you. What is it these people have. But the fact is that we've all got this in, in us. We have to find it.

We have to find a way. But what is most noticeable is that these people that are like that have got some sort of military background.

If you can imagine your life should be like driving in the dark. If you're driving your car in the dark, you look what's right in front of you.

You don't look to see what's behind you. It's gone.

You can only see as far as your beam will go. What's in the present moment, what's you have past, you don't even think about, you concentrate on what in front of you and that's how life should be. We should concentrate on that bit in front of us.

That's because you've only got so much energy. If you can get all your energy to one little bit. One second, one second, mate, one second.

Yeah, it's a bit like that, isn't it? That process of just living like that. Just concentrate on that little bit all the time.

Alan

Yeah, I do. I'm still at the. Cracking a lot of jokes because my legs have got complete spasticity now. I call myself a spaz and my mates get younger me, but you know, I am. It's got spasticity all over me medication box. When I get up in the mornings, it's. Sometimes I'm full of life and other days it's just swinging my legs off the bed and getting up is a, you know, it's dramatic but, but anyway, all I can do is thank you for opening up and telling us. You know, I'm full of admiration and I know people that know you that are kind of completely full of admiration, irrespective of whether you've climbed that Everest or you haven't and someone else has.

Jason

I went up mount Snowden a few years ago.

Alan

WoW, Everest next then.

We're going to leave it there because I am so, so happy with what you have told me for the readers.

I really appreciate you agreeing to take time out of your extremely busy diary to do this for me.

The whole point of this book is to help people, no matter what their problem is, to understand that they can seek help, but importantly, by hearing stories like yours, it highlights the fact that no matter how long the journey of recovery.

It’s worth it.

Chapter 29: James Ford (JT MOTIV)

James Ford is a successful mental health and addiction keynote speaker who has kindly agreed to be interviewed by me for the book.

James has an incredible story of which I could not write this intro until the interview was complete, I personally learned so much.

I clearly had a very negative view of alcoholics and drug users and I learned so much during this interview that completely stunned me, and it was noticeable for James as he was seeing my facial reactions to what he was saying.

Listening to James took me from anger to pity and wanting to give James a hug.

Alan:

Hi James, can we start at the beginning with your start in life as a child, this always help paint a picture for the readers, it helps for people to try and gauge as to whether the early years do dictate or direct us towards our negative choices.

James

Listen, great childhood. me and my older brother.

Didn't have a lot, it wasn't financially amazing, but we never wanted for anything. Loads of love, nice house, both parents worked, stayed together right through until see my dad passed away a few years ago. Great childhood. My brother had the same upbringing as me. We had a lot in terms of love and care and I've only got very fond memories of my childhood.

Yeah, it was amazing.

My first memory was at like two, three years old in a pram with a red canopy and she went yeah, that's right with the head that stuck out. Yeah, that's right. She said so I've got, I've got great fond memories of my past, my childhood.

Primary School was good, I loved school. Wasn't very academically clever but I attended did okay.

Secondary school was different, that's when things changed obviously hormones, emotions, peer pressure, all that came about. I was always in the in crowd at school. There's always an in crowd in school and I was always in that. Even though I was at the back of that queue. I was at the back of the in crowd, I was in it.

I did get bullied from people in the in crowd that were so called friends and from others as well and people outside school and I was very fearful as a child through the bullying really. I remember my parents had to take me, I had to pick up from school every day from sort of the second year in, first year I was fine Second year in through the bullying of outside my school day outside school.

They used to have to pick me up every single day and it was a good fifteen, twenty minutes from where we lived but I would always go to school early because I always thought that the bullies wouldn't get up early. So, I go to school early at half seven.

Again, I Wasn't academically clever in. In secondary school

I had visions of. I wanted to go in the navy, but that was in the RAF.

I always told the career teachers when they asked do what you want to do.

My reply was always the same, I want to be in the navy. I always said it for years; I'm going to go in the navy. I'm going to go in the navy. And obviously that didn't transpire.

Didn't really get many GCSEs.

My first taste of a drink was when on a Saturday night, you'd have to get a bottle of cider to share with Mum and Dad. He'd go, do you want a little glass? and he'd give me a little tumble of full at sort of twelve, thirteen. Same with my brother. Nothing extravagant.

They do the few drinks now and then and whatnot. And then I remember about fifteen in school. Obviously, a lot of my friends was. Was smoking weed and I. I've always had a bad chest. I've always had. I got diagnosed at nineteen with COPD under an immune deficiency, which I'll come on to later. But I've always suffered with asthma. They called isn't, but that's what they called it. So, I didn't really smoke or anything like that. And I tried. It wasn't my thing. Did the usual fifteen going on Parks, drinking.

I was drinking Miller. Four cans of Miller I'd have. And he and Alan. It didn't really light me up. Yeah. I wasn't really. I just did it because that's what the boys were doing. Yeah. But I didn't. Didn't really like it, so to speak. It didn't. Didn't light me up. Anyway. And then I remember leaving school. I didn't. I never went in the navy, as I've been saying for years. I thought. My dad said, you need to get a trade behind you. My dad was a joiner since he comes out the RAF. So, I said, well, I'll be a spark. I want to be electrician. So, I went and got an apprenticeship with a small Company, Family-owned company. Sixteen years old. I remember I was. We had Walkman's then.

My favourite band of all time were Oasis. So, they just come out. This was in ninety-five. Ninety-six. Yeah, ninety-five Ish. Oasis on me Walkman at work. I do a month in work and then a month in college, but the bullying kept going.

So, I left school, finished the bullying, went into college, started the bullying again, and it was even worse. It was really bad. Not only was it mental, but it was also physical as well, and again, it took a while. Took a right good few months, it took for me to sort of get friends with just two out of ten lads that sort of put a stop to the bullying from this guy who's an absolute tool

I started to enjoy my college and my work and stuff and I was earning money. I thought I was on ten pound a day. I thought I was absolutely loaded at fifty pound a week. Coming from doing paper rounds all through my school years, from being thirteen, I had three paper rounds from thirteen to sixteen, earning eighteen pound a week. And I always had money, I always saved and it was quite good and then when I got this job at fifty pound a week, I was like, I'm going to be loaded but the bullying took off and as I said before, that subsided after a good few months because I got in with these other two lads that put a stop to it. So, my dad said, James, now you're at work and you're at college, I need to take you to the pub for a proper pint, this was at sixteen. He said, but, you know, I'm not going to get you a pint of lager. You're going to have. I think it was either bitter or mild or something that. Mild and bitter, can't remember.

I don't know if that's it, but you can have mild. Pint of mild. Oh, my. It was rank. Alan and I drank it, but that never got me. So, I'm in the pub thinking, I'm an adult, drinking this pint with my dad in our local.

That ended up being our local for years but that never got me. What did get me was the flashing lights in the corner, the fruit machines and that was my first addiction. that's what got me. and I remember saying to my dad, have you got a couple of quid? and going on and loving it, loving the fruit machines and it quickly took hold.

At sixteen, I was getting paid on a Friday and I was putting all my money in the fruit machines in the arcades where I Lived and I would come back sometimes I would win. I remember this one time, it was a because every machine I played, I won. It was. It was like I had the Midas touch, and I remember coming out of there with one hundred and fifty pounds. So that's three weeks wages. I was absolutely over the moon. I didn't get the bus; I walked I had new Walkman on. I stopped at the shop; I got my dad a little bottle of whiskey because I could get served in this shop near me. I got my mum some chocolates. I go home and they were like, what are these for?

So, I was like, oh, I've just one of my fruit machines. And my dad's like, oh, be careful, son. Yeah, yeah, yeah, I'll be fine, dad. And then I remember for the next three weeks, then I lost all my wages for the next three weeks chasing what I'd done previous.

Always try to recapture the past when he had a good time and that comes out a little bit later with the drink and drugs, but it took me to some very, very dark places, the addiction of gambling very quickly because I remember at seventeen years old taking an overdose because me and my brother had had a row over putting my taxi money in the fruit machine and he had to pay and we had a massive row and I took an overdose and I got rushed to hospital, I was seventeen. The pills weren't life threatening. I just felt groggy for a good few days after and I remember my dad the next morning saying what happened? and I said oh, I'm fine. It sorts of got brushed under the carpet that one instance.

I finished my first-year college, passed with flying colours, went into my second year as an apprentice installing electric cables underground and stuff your heavy stuff HV & LV Cables and I moved colleges from Stockport to Openshaw College and I just passed my driving test. So, there I was in me mum and dad bought. I bought my own car; I bought my first car off of my dad.

I wasn't into drinking at all. So, what I used to, but I was really into the fruit machine still didn't go in the bookies or anything.

I remember I would drive round to different pubs and I would buy lime and soda because it was twenty pence and then I could put all my money in the fruit machines and I'd win and go to another pub, win and go to another, or lose or whatever and this went on for a while and it took me to some very, very dark places where I was putting all my money in.

I was thinking, what am I doing? and then I remember it. Eighteen and a half, nineteen, I picked up drink again because I never drank. On the eighteenth birthday, my mum and dad threw me a massive party with all my friends and family, and I was in bed sober at half ten.

Everyone's having a great time till four in the morning.

Drink Just didn't do anything for me, and I remember at eighteen and a half I left being electrician and I went working at Morrisons as a fishmonger at eighteen and a half. I know it's just. It's a very strange transition, but that's what I did.

I was working with an older chap there, still friends with him to this day, even though he's in a quite a bad way but anyway, that's another story and he introduced me to cocaine.

I remember I'd mither him for a good few months to give us some and he kept saying, no, no, no, because I was, at that time I was going through my diagnosis because they didn't know what was wrong with me because they'd realized it wasn't asthma. So, I was having all these tests of why I kept getting poorly. It ended up that I've got severe COPD and I've got a rare immune deficiency. and that's what I was diagnosed with at nineteen.

At this time, I was getting tested and diagnosed. I was asking for drugs from my friend and he kept saying, no, your poorly. We don't know what's wrong with you, I'm not giving it you and ended up after a couple of months of me mithering and he gave in and they had my first line and it was on a Friday night, it was dark, rainy, the four of us, it was. Four of us always went out. We just had a massive fight in the. Our local pub with these lads that had come down from another town, and I asked him for come Charlie and he went, yeah.

So, I had my first line ever at nineteen, eighteen and a half. Sorry. and I knew Alan from that point. I was hooked.

I know that because that was on a Friday night. I then bought a bag of coke Saturday, Sunday, Monday, Tuesday, Wednesday, every single night for Five days. And I remember on the Wednesday, I remember I had a very old Sony Ericsson phone, a Big thick thing. And I remember at two in the morning, chopping a line up off the back of my phone in bed and I remember thinking, is this normal? People must do this. It's not just me. This must be normal. This is what everybody does that takes coke.

I remember it, it got me because I would. I would be sniffing coke. Not drinking at the time just sniffing coke four or five times a week, easy. Getting in debt. It was when it was. It was the dearest it's ever been coke. So, I was getting in loads of debt for it. And I remember within four months I had a massive breakdown in work because I was constantly sniffing, not drinking and a massive breakdown. I went. Went on the sick for two months.

Now, in those four months before I had my breakdown, I would walk in, I was the instigator, and I would walk into work at six in the morning where we would decorate the fish counter with all the fish and it was freezing because they're all packed with ice, and I would walk in with an eighth of coke and I'd dangle it in my friend's face and he would get quite upset, he'd be quite angry because he couldn't help himself either. Yeah, he couldn't say no, like me. So, his words were, you're an absolute wanker but what we'll do is let's get some food first. So, we've eaten for the day. Yeah. and then we'll get on it and that's what we did. So, we stole some sandwiches and some drinks and crisps from the sandwich bar next door at Morrisons, at them in the back at six in the morning we'd have our first line at say, seven and we'd be on it all day, working till three and then we'd go to the pub and carry on. and that was in those four months, and I would do this a lot? Anyway, I had a breakdown, was off work for two months. I remember my mum Saying, you've got a chemical imbalance. I think they knew what I was up to, but they didn't know the extent of it and I remember my mum saying, you need to go to the doctors. You see how she got to the point of the doctors. I'd be nineteen, still living at home. I just got with an older bird. My first proper girlfriend who was nine years older than me. And I used to stay at her house, but I'd go on benders. I'd go on weekend benders Friday to Sunday and my mum would come in my room on a Monday morning, and she'd say I'd be in bed or just getting up and she'd go, be about half, about nine o' clock, she'd go, you, you're not going to work again. So, I'd say, no, Mum. She'd go, I can't believe you've rang in sick. Why can't you be like your brother? Why can't you go out on a Friday and Saturday night and then come and have your Sunday dinner with us and then go work on a Monday? Why have you got to go out on a Friday and we don't see you till Sunday night? and at that time I said the most honest answer I caught at that time and I just said, I don't know, Mum. I don't know why I keep doing what I'm doing, and it didn't at that time and that's when she'd say, I'm going to take you to the doctors. You've got a chemical imbalance. You need to rebalance your yin and yang.

So, she took me to the doctors, and I tell the doctor what's happening but not the truth of course, a brief explanation of what I was up to, wouldn't go into too much detail and the doctor would go, like a lot of doctors do that don't understand. You're depressed. So let me sign you off, let me give you some antidepressants and here's some beta blockers. There you go. You'd be fine. Right? So not only was I then taking coke and drinking, I was also on antidepressants and beta blockers at nineteen to rebalance this chemical thing that I've got that my mum thinks I had.

This became a continual cycle. Three out the four weekends I would go on my benders and don't know why.

I moved in with this girl that was nine years older than me and I was still working at Morrisons, but not as a fishmonger anymore because I thought that guy was the problem that I work with. So, I went and did Nights. That's going to help me, sleep all day, work through the night. That, that's. That will fix me. You see, I was always all over the years I was always looking at external things that are going to fix me inside. So, I would do stuff like change my job, change where I live, change the misses Go to the gym, not go to the gym. They were all outside circumstances that I thought would fix my internal condition of why I drank and used. So, it ended up that I was causing my mum and dad loads of grief at nineteen and a half. And I moved in with this girl.

I've been with her not even a year and she got pregnant and we had a child. When she got pregnant, straight away I thought, I'm fixed. Course the responsibility of having a child is going to fix me. How could it not going to be all right and for the nine months as my partner was pregnant.

I left Morrisons because again I thought it's the problem. So, I left Morrisons and I went working in a sales job. I went working for a charity and it was selling tickets for a raffle in a shop doorway and it was great money, was earning really, good money. For the late nineties, I was earning four, five hundred pound a week cash. Now for the nineties, that was great money just by standing and selling tickets in a shop doorway and I never touched a drug in nine months as my missus was pregnant. I drank a few times, but I never touched a drug in nine months, and I held it down and that made me think, I've not got a problem ever, because if I can stop on my own accord, I've not got a problem. and then my daughter was born, Charlotte, in the year two thousand. And I thought, well, this is it, this is it. I've not done it for nine months; I'm not going to do it now.

I'm all right. I ended up leaving and got this charity job because it was a little bit, dodgy, I wasn't naughty. The charity got money, which was fine, but the people that owned the company were absolutely wadded. Anyway, I left and I remember my misses Saying, do you think it's time, James, you need to go and get a proper job? And I said, yeah.

What about this here? Bank of Scotland Telesales, a company car after six months. Yeah, that sounds mega offer. Went for the interview, got the job and I always. I've never been in the call centre before nearby and of course I'm not really drinking and using it at this time. I'm thinking I'm holding it down and I've got it together and then I remember walking in, my daughter was. I think my daughter was about eight months old. No, she about five months old when I got this job and I was very good at the job, very good at sales that have been in my whole background for my whole life.

The drinking culture and the using culture in a call centre was off the scale. I'd never seen anything like it. These people drank and used coke like me; they loved it. They were up until four or five in the morning in people's kitchens and we were always planning nights out, trips out. That's what we did. But they could do something that I couldn't do. When they woke up on a Sunday morning, they felt groggy. They had a shower and got something to eat and tidied the house and chilled out ready for work on the Monday. They had that choice to stop. They could just say NO; I'm not doing that today. I've got responsibilities. I have got that choice. I would wake up and I would have this obsession, this compelling to drink, to drink or use or whatever to carry it on, to try and capture the great moments of the past. Whether it be the night before because it was a great night, or a few weeks before or whatever it may be.

I was about twenty, my daughter was just born. So yeah, twenty, twenty-one, she'd just been born in two thousand. And I'm not saying it was bad all the time. I had some bad times in drinking controls, like really, sad times. But I also had some amazing times as well that ended up in some amazing places.

These benders, these continued for years. So, as I said for nine months as she was pregnant, I never used. I drank now and then. I then got in this call centre.

Everyone was like me, or so I thought. And my drinking and using went off the scale. I went back on it quicker than anything.

I could never really put it down to. I needed to stop me drinking and using. But it was all fun. It was with the boys. It's what everybody did. But it got to the point where it was every weekend, I used to cause rows with the misses on Purpose so I could do one for the weekend. Spending money that wasn't mine, spending bill money that was hers, just being an absolute nuisance and then it ended up that I had another idea, Alan, this one's going to fix me this time because obviously I'm a bit lost now at twenty-three. I'll get my own place now. I already had a house with the misses and my daughter and her and my missus's first son, he was about ten. So already at that house, already had my own. I need my own little pad because that's going to save me. So, I went and bought a house. I went and bought a cottage flat, a two story. I went about the top flat; this was in two thousand three and that was when the days of my drinking and using when the worst they've ever been because I know we've got a lot of digital stuff with the phones now and what not and People know where you are and what you're doing. Wasn't like that for me in two thousand three. Phone calls were texting and ringing, that was it. And I could quite easily go missing for a week.

My family would think I was at work, and I would ring in work and say I've got a chest infection. You see, I would play on my illness a lot in my drinking and using days and they would say no problem, James, get well soon, we'll see you next week and that. And I used to go, brilliant, that. Give me a week. Then drinking and using, I never left the house. I used to get it posted through the letterbox every day and I would, I would, when I'd. I'd buy loads of, of beer and whiskey and when it had gone, I would be petrified to leave the house to go and get more. Absolutely beside myself, shaking and shivering, thinking, oh, something's going to happen And then I scuttle to the shop which was only down the road, it's only five minutes down the road, buy as much as I can with the money that I had and then back in and then stay for another two or three days in the flats watching all the usual Jeremy Kyle, This morning, all the usual rubbish that's on telly in the mornings, drinking and using and I remember when my brother rang me on a Monday morning and I'd been on a bender from the Friday.

He said, where are you? and I said I'm, I'm in the flat now. So, I said, no.

You need to, James, you need, you need to tow the party line, and I'm thinking, tow the party line.

There's no party going on. It's a Monday morning at half nine. I'm drinking warm whiskey from the bottle, sniffing Coke off the mantelpiece, watching Jeremy Kale, thinking, my life's not that bad. There's no party going on. I'm on my own. There's no party. I don't know why I keep doing what I do.

You need help. I know we need help. And it was always, doctors, doctors, go to the doctors. Now. By this time, I was twenty-three, twenty-four, and I wasn't even going on the work dos anymore and stuff because it was just an absolute liability and it ended up that 90% of what I drank was from twenty-four to twenty-five and a half years of age. It was just bad. I never left the house. I would drink during working hours and go in, work for a couple of hours and then say, I'm not well, and go back. It was just my life revolved around drinking, drugs. Everything I did, everywhere I went, you see, drink.

Drink dictated what I did in my life. It told me when I got up, it told me when I went to bed, it told me who I hung around with, it told me how much money I had. It dictated everything. It ruled everything, and everything evolved around it and a new deep down that I needed to do something about it, but I didn't know what. I didn't know how. And I used to say, quite openly, I'll be dead by the time I'm twenty-five. And I'd say that to my parents, well, it's all right. I'm going to be dead by the time I'm twenty-five and twenty-five came and ended up that I was in a real bad way, on my own in a bad, bad way and I remember there was a family friend that had been to the recovery rooms of Alcoholics Anonymous, and she was about ten years sober and I remember thinking, I don't know what to do. I don't know where to go. But obviously this lady did because she was sober. So, I knocked on the door. It was actually a Friday night. I'd been on a bender that week or stopped on the Monday and Tuesday, so I knocked on her door on the Friday, and I said, can you take me to a meeting? And she said, yeah, I'll just grab my coat. so I went, what, now? You're going to take me now? Yeah, let's go right this second. I was like, whoa, whoa, whoa. I didn't mean now. She says, no, come on, get in the car, we'll go. And that was my first taste of my first recovery meeting at twenty-five and a half.

Alan

So, what. What was the moment that you decided to do that? Were you at your lowest point at this stage?

James

Yes, I was at the lowest point of my life at that point. I'd never been that low before, So, you see, going through what I call it my drinking drug career, Alan. So, when I'm going through it, I used to have these. These thoughts off.

When I lose my license, I'll stop drinking. I lost my license twice and then I would change. Well, if I lose my flat, I'll stop drinking. If I lost my misses, I'd stop drinking. And I always put conditions on it. If I. Every time I. I'd lose whatever I said I wouldn't. I would just keep moving the goal posts. So, at twenty-five and a half, when I went into recovery, that was the worst I've ever been because all the goal posts had been moved and I was like, yeah, I'm stuck now. I'm stuck. I was absolutely stuck and I didn't know nowhere else to go. So, yeah, definitely.

Alan:

Sorry, can I ask you a question? Did you make promises to people that you're going to stop, people that cared about you and just break the promises all the time? Is that what you mean by moving a goalpost?

James

Yeah. Yes and no.

Alan:

Or were you doing it in your own mind?

James

I was doing it in my own mind, but with the promises.

So, on a Monday, when that conversation I've just had where my mum said, why can't you be like your brother? And I said, and he used to say. She said, why can't you? I said, I don't know. That was the only stance. Now, at that time, I would say to my mum, I promise, I promise I'll stop. And. And I meant it. If you would have put me on a lie detector test at that point, I would have passed that lie detector.

Jeremy Kyle would have come out and said, he's got a full house, he's passed. Yeah. Because I was telling the truth. I meant it. I'm never doing it again. That promise was broken. On the Thursday when I would finish work, my friend did go, James, are you coming for a bottle of bud? And it's not like I forget what's happened on the Monday with me mum. I just go, all right, I can have the one. You see, my mind convinces me that it won't be like it was last Time. And I'll just have the one. I was constantly making sweet promises. The worst person that I did it to and kept breaking was my daughter. For the first ten years of her life, I wasn't present. I was physically, but nowhere near emotionally present with my daughter. Not one bit. And people say that's because you chose drinking drugs. No, I never chose drinking drugs because if I had a choice, I around drinking drugs.

If I had a choice, I would have chosen my daughter. Yeah, that proves that I do not have a choice. I'm not. I'm not a social degenerate. I'm not choosing drinking drugs over my daughter. I don't have a choice around that. I'm just geared up. I'm. My default setting is drinking and drugs. But my mind sees the difference Says my mind convinces me every single time that I can just have the one every time. My mind never says, right, you're going to go out and you're going to get. Absolutely. It always started with one, always. And I'll end there. And it never did. I'd say once out of a hundred, I'd have a couple of bottles of bud, A couple of pints, and then I would stop for the rest of the night because I had some social event that was very important, but I weren't happy. I would make sure that every. Everybody there wasn't happy at that social event as well, because I wasn't drinking. Very, very selfish. Okay.

Alan:

So, we know what addiction took from you, which was your daughter, I would assume, some friends. And your relationship with your mum and dad and your brother was struggling. So, you start the process now of getting clean. What is the process of getting clean? I know you've made the first step and the lady took you to Alcoholics Anonymous. What actually happens when you walk in for the first time, just so people reading this know what to expect.

James

I didn't know what to expect, I had no expectations. And when I walked in, I was greeted with very, very lovely people. I walked the walk. I'd walked and come through the other side. So, I knew that there was something in it and a new experience from my friend being over ten years. So, I walked in. The people were amazing But You see, it’s not just about going to meetings and getting a support network. The support network is massively important. But there's certain stuff that you need to do in the AA rooms to change your mindset, change your behaviours. If you Just go to meetings and tell your story. Nothing's going to change. If you change Nothing, then Nothing changes. All I'm doing is going to a meeting and telling my stories. I have to physically sit down with somebody that's been before me. And we have. It's called the Big Book. It's Alcoholics Anonymous. We call it the Big Book. It's not big. It's just a normal book. That's what. It's just what it's called.

So, we have a book that we read together with what's called a sponsor, and they take you through the twelve Step Fellowship, the twelve Step program of Alcoholics Anonymous. Now, this was written in nineteen thirty-nine, so it's been going for nearly ninety years and has saved Millions and millions, tens of millions of people and their families from the darkness, but when I got there, Alan, I wasn't ready. I only know this reflecting back because for the first four months, all I did was what. There was two people that. What happens is you walk in, you sit in a circle most of the time, and somebody will just open the meeting. That's like me. And people share their experience, strength and hope.

I remember my first meeting; One guy said, James, just keep coming to meetings, share your story, and you'll get better. And I thought, well, I can do that because my favourite subject is me, so I can talk about me, that I can do that, no problem.

Then this other chap straight after said, James, my experience is a little bit different, my friend. Of course, you've got to come to meetings and share that. That's part of it, because you're getting a support network in place. So, I had said, that book over there, he said in there he's outlined is a program of recovery, and its what changes our behaviour and our mindset. And we need to do that to have it. What's called a psychic change. It's all in the book. He said, but it's going to take a bit of hard work and you'll have to find a sponsor and go through it, and I'll take you a good six weeks. But once you've done that, you'll get given a brand-new life. You'll be a different person. Trust me. And when he finished his share, in my head I went, well, that sounds like hard work and the other guy, I can just come to meetings and share my story And I'll get out.

According to him, I'll get better. Well, I can do that. So that's the option I chose. I'll just keep coming to meetings. I won't do any of that twelve-step work. I don't need to. My brain again convinces me because at the end of the day, my brain, my, my head does not want me in an AA meeting. It doesn't and I will come on a bit late. Alcoholism is an illness. It's a two-fold illness recognized by the World Health Organization as an illness.

So, it takes work. And I didn't really want to work. I just thought I'll come and share and it for four months I was dry. I never picked up a drink or drug in four months, and I did these meetings and I kept sharing Everything I'm doing and I picked up after four months because nothing changed.

I was still cheating on the misses, dealing drugs, lying, cheating. I was doing all that. I was just not drinking and using. Four months picked up and then every time I picked up over the years it got that little bit worse. A little bit worse, a little bit worse. It just carved another bit away from me. Chipping away, chipping away. And I ended up being in recovery. So, from twenty-six to thirty-one for five years, I messed about. I was in and out, in and out.

Alan

These people that you sit with, they're experienced enough to know that you are talking and some of them must be looking at you and thinking that you are lying, and you're on it.

James

One hundred percent

Alan:

All right. Okay. Do they pull you on it? Are they comfortable enough pulling you on it? Or do they just not listen? And out can see in their demeanour they're not really listening because they know you're not genuine.

James

Correct. So, I would never, I've never ever drank and used in a meeting. I know some people have. I've never drank and used in a meeting. People that I know, people that drink and use and go to a meeting. That's the worst place I'd want to be. I want to be in some casino or in some guy's house or something with a load of lads.

Alan:

Standing in the kitchen talking bollocks with strangers who are suddenly your best mates.

James

Yes. I definitely don't want to be in a meeting.

When I said that People would suss me out. Yeah. They would know just the way I was speaking. And I wasn't putting in the work. We call them the old timers.

They've seen thousands of me coming in all the Designer Gear being the wide boy and all that. And they think he's not ready.

They never say it to me. They would never. Nobody ever comes up to me and go, you're not ready. You. They would come and just try and help, but they know in the back of the mind that I was going to go back and fuck it all up again.

I'd hit another rock bottom at twenty-five, and I did four months, then picked up. Did two months, then picked up. I kept making all these excuses and felt that I was too young.

I think the average age in AAA at the time was fifty-five. Okay. So, I was twenty-six. I remember an old guy coming over to me and he said, James, he said, if you get this now at twenty-six, you can have the best life. And me being me, my thinking had not changed. I thought, hang on a minute, you've had twenty years of drinking on me. As if that's a good thing. Yeah, no, he's had twenty years of hell on. But I didn't see it as that.

It was New Year's Eve. Sorry, the day before New Year's Eve, two thousand six, and I'd gone back drinking. And again, I thought, I think we'd had a great Christmas, two thousand six. And I thought, right, I'm going to start an argument. Because I had me flat that was being sold and it was empty apart from a sofa and a big box TV and a DVD player and loads of DVD's. So, I'm going to cause a row. I'll walk to the shop, get a couple of bottles of whiskey, get a taxi to be flat, job done, I'm on my own watching DVD's, I'm going to get on it. And I did that for three days. And all I kept doing was scuffling to the shop, buying another bottle of whiskey and coming back. And I did it for three days. And I remember this is in going from two thousand six into the beginning of two thousand seven.

I remember a knock on the door, Alan, I woke up or come to. I had a white sofa, let me tell you, weren't white. After three days, I come to and I'd look at the side of me and I'd see a bottle of whiskey at the side with half of it gone. And I take the biggest glug I could without being sick and it'd give me them Shivers that I would go down my neck and then I'd put it down and it had knocked me out again. And I did that for three days. And I remember on New Year's Day, about half past eight in the morning, nine o' clock in the morning, there was a knock at the door and I jumped up and I looked out the window because I was on the second floor, my mum's car's outside. So, I ran downstairs, open the door, and there she is with four bin bags. And she said she doesn't want you anymore. She said,

That's, that's it, you're done. Happy New Year, son. And I remember we had a quick chat. She saw the state of the flat. There was bottles everywhere, there was Chinese cartons everywhere, because I'd had that on the first day. And I remember she gave me a kiss and she went. Walked out. And honestly, with hand on heart, I wanted to say, mom, help me. Please help me. Everything I just wanted to. To say, help.

Alan:

Why didn't you? Hey, why didn't you?

James:

Because I had fifteen quid in my back pocket.

Alan:

All right, okay. So, you would value help, but only under your conditions and when it suited you.

James:

You were at the bottom; I was at the bottom, and I really wanted to ask her for help. And I remember looking out the window, she'd left. I remember looking out the window about fifteen minutes after she'd shut the door and her car was still outside and there she was, crying. Yeah, and that's the point where I was like, just go, just, just go outside now, James, just say, need help? And I thought, well, no, because you've got fifteen quid in your back pocket. That'll get you about four or five pints. And the pubs open at eleven o'. Clock. You've got two hours to wait. I had nothing left in the house and that's exactly what I did.

Alan:

You're annoying me. Here, you're annoying me with this story, you selfish bastard.

James:

I am awful. I am horrendous. Yeah, I am horrendous. Sorry, I'll rephrase. Alan. I was horrendous.

Alan:

I know, I know.

James:

But, but, but, but this is, this is, this is the thing with the illness of addiction. I was so wrapped up in, in, in me. I didn't, I wasn't arsed about anything. I wasn't washing, wasn't showering, wasn't brushing my teeth, wasn't shaving, didn't give a fuck About anything. As long as I had my drink.

I Remember walking to the pub at quarter to eleven, eleven o', clock, all the boys should come in. Not my boys, just all the boys would come and saying, great night last night, did it. I remember I got a pint and a double whiskey and honestly, hand on heart, I was shaking like a hitting because I was going into alcoholic withdrawals. And I bought it and I sat down, Alan, and I never even took the head off it. It never touched my lips and the shakes stopped. They just stopped because I knew my body knew what was going in. And I stopped for about a minute and a half, two minutes. It just stopped and I drank it. And I remember after the first double whiskey in the first pint, I remember the ego rebuild. I remember. I remember sitting back in the booth of this pub that I was at on my own. I remember sitting back, going, everything's going to be all right.

Dead chilled. I went, dead chilled. And I had my three or four pints and he had four quid left or something.

I walked home, got my last few cans and I remember I rang my partner who had just kicked me out at about four o', clock, and I went, can you come for me, please? I had no more money, no food, no nothing. And she came and got me and she went, you know what you need to do? You need to go back to the rooms of

AA. So, I did, and I went back on the seventh, the second of January, two thousand seven, which was my dad's birthday. And my parents sort of knew because I went. They went, are you having a drink? I went, can I just have a Pepsi? And they also looked at you each other like that they knew. Anyway, that was that Up until that point, two thousand seven was the best year of my life. And I'm going to explain why.

So, second of January 2007 was the start of the best year of my life up to that date. And obviously the dealing had gone, and the cheating had gone and. And I thought, no, I need to do something that I've never done before. And I've learned later on in life that if you do something that you've never done before, you'll get changes that you've never had before. Yeah. So, I thought, I need to do this. So, I did. And I said there was. Dude. All I concentrated on in two thousand seven was three things in this order. Number one was recovery, first and foremost. The second one was my family. And the third one was work. I didn't care what I am, I didn't go to the gym, I didn't do anything else apart from those three things in that order.

I remember I was working at the AA, funny enough, ironically, at the Automobile association, on the phones, giving breakdowns. Mad. Anyway, I remember I was working there now. I joined there six months previous, but when I went missing for three days over New Year, I was employed by them and I've got in that much trouble, so I went AWOL over the New year when I was drinking in my flat, I thought, when I walk in in the new year, I'm going to get sacked because I was on my last warning, you're going to get a curly finger, and sacked. So, second of January, went and saw my dad for his birthday. Everyone was a bit puzzled why I wasn't drinking. They had an idea, went back in work on the third and I thought, you're going to walk in, James, and they're going to say your sacked. And I walked in and I was met by a guy. My manager was a girl and I was met by this guy and he went, you're James, I said, I am. I'm your new manager. So I says, right.

He 'ent, your old manager. Ha' gone to another department now. I've heard loads about you and it's not good, but I'm not about that. Let me. You start afresh and draw a line in the sand and then we'll see how we get on. Yeah? I was like, thank you, thank you, thank you. Because I've just, I've just dodged a bullet again. Don't mess it up this tim', James.

I just threw myself into recovery then my family spending as much time as I could in work. And I remember after a month my manager would we become really, really good friends. I remember after a month of me always turning up on time, staying late, dressing to impress, helping other people, I had no drink or drugs to suppress my capabilities. So, my sales pattern was next level. And I could sell sand to the Arabs, as the saying goes. I was doing very, very well. I remember after a month, six weeks, my manager came over, he looked over my shoulder and I'm reading a book. And he went, what's that you're reading? And I told him it's the Alcoholics Anonymous big book. And he got a bit sort of nervous. Oh, oh, okay. So, I said, it's fine. And he went. His words were, can we do anything as a company to help you? And I was totally shocked at the moment, then I said No but if there is anything, I'll let you know. And he said, we're here to help.

Now this is before all the mental health came in and all that. Like twenty years later. Even then, companies had stuff in place to go, how can we help you? And in that year, I focused on those three things that I've said before. And in that year, my recovery. I hit a year sober on the second of Jan, two thousand eight. I won two awards from the AA because I've made him the most. I was number one salesman. I was number one the whole country. And I made them the most profit out the whole country. They were using my sales calls in their training centre. This is how it should be done.

So, everything was going amazingly, and my family life was incredible and I was having the best year of my life up until that point but inside I was like every day was a struggle. I would go to meetings, I'd get a sponsor, which is what they told me to do, And I did something, as I said before, that I've not done before, which was a twelve-step program of recovery. I went through it as it's outlined in the book, and I changed. I didn't, I was given a brand-new life and I changed. I wasn't that person anymore. I was, I was a brand-new James then in two thousand eight, I was a year sober. It was one of the best days ever. I remember the feeling. It was incredible. And I thought, right, I'm going to start implementing a few of the little bits to my life now because.

I put on loads of weight and I had to start ironing me T shirts with a wok. So, I thought, I'm going to go to the gym. So, I joined the Gym on my birthday, on my AA birthday, my sobriety birthday, second of January, two thousand eight. And Alan, within four months, I picked up. I picked up again after four months. And what happened in those four months was I joined the gym. I got addicted to the gym. I was going to the gym five times a week, and I was only doing the recovery rooms twice a week. So that what I said before about having recovery number one, family number two, work number three, the gym was number one and recovery was number two. And that experience showed me that if you put anything in front of recovery, you'll lose it all.

So, after four months, I picked up and I was at the Ricky Hatton fight when he very first came out in his fat suit at the Etihad Stadium. And I remember I never drank, but all day I was convinced that I would and I was mentally saying please don't drink, please don't drink.

It was on me. Go 'n, have a drink. Have a drink. Have a drink. This voice in my head, go on, have a drink. Have a drink. And I remember, I got through the whole night, got in a taxi, got back to my house. I remember sitting down with a big sigh of relief.

I've done it. And the friend that I was with pulled out a bag of coke and I looked at him and I just said, I'll have one of them. Just like that, instantly, sixteen months down the drain, I'll have one of them. And this, this person never said, no, no, no, don't do that. His words were, yes, James is back.

So, during that time, everything you got, back when you had that good year with your daughter, your family, etc, just went in one fell swoop of seeing a bag of shovel. Okay, see, I'm trying to understand it. And that's why it's important for the book. People need to understand it. They need to understand.

Alan:

The voice that you mention can only come be described by someone like yourself who has the lived experience to tell them that it might not just be them. Because I've never been in your position, so I don't understand it, but it's fascinating to listen to. It really is.

James:

That's why I could see you getting a little bit angry, because it's frustration.

Alan:

Really? It's because you've got your life and you're throwing it away. and because I can't understand it, that's why I need to listen to it. I'm not. I'm not angry. I feel sad for you because people that have not had it just want to say, well, why'd you do it? You know what I mean?

People like me, just want to shout STOP. It's as simple as that. Just stop.

Having said that, I've been a fat all my life, and I only lost weight when I become ill.

If I said to someone, why don't you stop smoking? They go, well, why don't you stop eating? It's not that simple, is it? But, yeah, so I'm not angry. It's just frustrating to listen to because I want you to stop. I want you to get to the part of the story where you can tell us it's all worked out well and all that stuff. But to get there, we need to hear the low parts.

James:

Yeah, definitely. So, I ended up picking up, and I was. The next morning, I learned I was fuming, absolutely fuming. And I remember going to a meeting the next day and seeing my sponsor at the time and. And he said, were you back to square one? And I was like, no, I'm not. I was fuming. No, I'm not. He went, no, you are. I said, no. Drink was my problem. Drugs was never my problem. And he went, James, you're back to day one. And I was fuming. So, I did what I did best. And I fucked him off, you're not being in my life then Again, a little bit of a slippery slope, because within two months. And this is how baffling, and powerful the disease of alcoholism is, the illness of alcoholism is, because There's no thought and within two months, I picked up everything again. And this is how quick it was. I was out with my friend at the time who gave me the line of coke when I asked, I asked for it. And we'd been out driving about, listening to music. Gets back in. My parents were in bed. I sat in my dad's seat, looked down, there's half a bottle of white wine. And I just picked it up and drank it. I didn't even think. I just picked it up and drank it. And my friend actually just went, no, you haven't and from that point then, that was it. That was middle of two thousand eight, from that point then till I finally gave in at august twenty ten. So that was like two years. And I massively went downhill Within three months.

Yeah. I was in and out of the AA rooms and then Christmases I were really bad because I was just drinking from seven in the morning and regrettably my daughter was Seeing it all.

I Didn't sell me flat, I still had it. So, I used to disappear there and I would. I was constantly for those two years, Alan, building the structure up and then pulling it down. Whether that was within a week, three weeks, three months. My parents had heard all the false promises again with my daughter, my partner at the time, my parents, my brothers, my sister in laws. He's got it this time, James has got it, he's on it. Bang. Something happens three weeks later, bang, I pick up and then I go on a weeklong bender.

In those two years everything got worse and worse and worse.

I ended up as the number one salesman at the AA to having to resign before I got sacked because I was not turning up.

Within months I was turning up late. I wasn't top salesman anymore. I was causing trouble. I was dealing drugs in there. Within months I'd gone right back downhill worse than I was when I first went in. And it ended up that I had to go.

We are now in two thousand nine and it ended up that I had to go into treatment. First time I'd been in a rehab centre and I was still employed by the AA at that time and I was on the sick and I was in rehab.

My parents paid for the rehab for me. I lasted five weeks and jumped out the wind fell and climbed out the window and went. Went to this, this other girl's house I was seeing because I was always having different girls in different ports and stuff. And I remember going to hers and I came out of treatment. I think it was about two months later, two and a bit. I remember leaving treatment going, I don't need treatment. Going back to the rooms, getting with this girl, this other girl, not the, not the mother of my child, some other girl. And I remember I remember I got six months sober and it's up. Just picked up again randomly just picked up in a shop.

This was in two thousand nine. And then. So, I didn't have a job because I had to resign from the AA. I didn't get any employment then for two years my uncle would try and help me and he would take me on jobs where he was electrician and because I'd done a bit of electrician in the past, he'd come and say that on this job for me and I chiselled wall boxes out and pull cables through and all bits and he tried, he just tried and helped me and it ended up that in the last year of my drinking and using I just, everything just chipped away.

So, it ended up that I wasn't with the mother of my daughter. I got rid of this girl who had moved in with me, tried to get back with the mother of my daughter. She was having none of it. She stopped me seeing my daughter because she said, she said you can't even look after yourself so you're not seeing your daughter. So, I ended up not seeing my daughter for nine months.

Didn't see her once.

My brother and my sister in laws all disowned me because I was a nuisance. The last two people that, that were with me would be mum and dad. Dad was quite frail; he was only out late fifties but he was very poorly. The illness that I've got of the COPD, my dad's got exactly the same. My dad died of it in twenty nineteen, he got a massive infection, and he passed away in mine, in my mum's arms.

So, he's very frail and very poorly. And I remember they were the last two people that disowned me. So, I was unemployable. No family, no daughter, nowhere to live, no job, nothing. Just got on benefits, or was it? Yeah, I think I just started to get a few benefits and I was just going missing for days and turning up at three in the morning, hospital. I'm thinking my mum saying pick me up, I was a mess. And then it ended up that.

I went on this bender, this last bender, the bender to end all benders. I didn't know that at the time. And I remember I've been, I've been on a drinking session, and I remember I rang my mum again at three in the morning in hospital. She came and picked me up and she took me home. I remember waking up the next morning at ten to eight and going downstairs. Now the usual scenario with this was I would go downstairs, the front door would be locked and I'd say let me out because I needed a drink, let me out. And my parents would go no, no, they're there, James, come on. And they'd put me back in bed with food and, and like water, a little bit like train spotting when they used to lock each other in the room and stuff so they could do the rattle. And that's what they do for three days. And then after three days there's no alcohol in your system. It's physically impossible to crave alcohol after three Days, because it's not in your system, okay?

It's all up here. It's a mental obsession that, that people think it's a craving. It's not. So, after there's a lot me in the room for three days, no more alcohol in my system. Did send me back to the recovery rooms of AA.

This particular time, Alan, I've tried the door, it's locked. I've turned on to my mum and I've gone, let me out as I always did. And she handed me the keys and she said, there you go, James. See you later. She said, me and your dad, we're done. Go and sleep under the viaducts with all the other winos. She says, bye. And again, this is the second time it's happened in my life. It's never happened. After this I really wanted to go.

No, help me. I don't. I don't know where. When I drink, I don't know where I end up. I don't know what I do, I don't know where they end up. It's very, very messy. And I wanted to say, help me. But again, I had sixty quid and I thought, and I actually thought, how many, how many cans of special brew can I get with sixty quid? And I went on this last bender that lasted eleven days How hard would it have been for my mum and dad to do that to the son? Can't even comprehend it. And off I went. And I did buy me four Cans of special brew. And I sat in a park on, I think it was around the seventeenth of August, two thousand and ten.

Red hot, boiling, mums and dads, taking the kids to the park. I'm sat in a corner with a big Henry Lloyd coat on, sweating, back out drinking this special brew, thinking, what am I doing? I couldn't. Once I started, then I was on it, I forgot sixty quid, and ended up going to this other girl's house who was like me, who drank like me. And we bought a bottle of vodka each. Now I only took the neck off. We both took the neck off the bottle of vodka each. All of a sudden, this girl went nuts, totally crazy and absolutely battered me all over the flat and I mean annihilated me. My eye was like a football. I was black and blue, I was bleeding. It ended up that the caretaker of the, the flat she was living took me to hospital.

I got bandaged up, got seen to, I came out the hospital, got in a taxi and went straight back to the girl's house because I knew she still has got the bottle of vodka there. And I stayed with her there for another three days, even though she just absolutely annihilated me. And then it ended up that. She kicked me out, because that's what happens. I get kicked out of these places and ended up that she kicked me out, ended up sleeping rough people, sofas. All the money had gone and more. I borrowed more.

I was done and I was turning yellow. I've not washed, I've not eaten properly. I've not done anything. All I've done for eleven days was drink. I Don't even think I used any drugs in them eleven days because it was too expensive. And I just wanted to put all my money into drink. And I remember on the eleventh day, I was broken. And I rang my mom, this was the twenty sixth of august, twenty ten. And I rang my mom and I said, help me. And she said, come home. You've got one more chance.

That was my last ever drink.

So, I came home and they did what they do. They put me in bed, but they didn't put me in my bed in my bedroom. I was too bad.

I ended up. I ended up going in my mum and dad's bed. My dad stayed downstairs. And for a grown man at thirty-one to be crying to his mum, begging her for another drink.

She said, I haven't got any. And she had. She had. Because you can't. You can't. It's not. It's not very good to stop drinking suddenly because you can go into what's called the delirium tremors, the DTs, where you. You have seizures. You can have what's called an alcoholic seizure. It's not good at all. But there was nothing I could do because I knew that if I started, I wouldn't stop. So, I had to stop. I had to just cut all ties, not drink. So, I spent three days in my mum's bed with her cradling me at thirty-one, both of us crying our eyes out. And the one thing that I was begging her for was the one thing that she knew was killing me, we both knew was killing me. And it ended up that those three days were the worst three days of my life. I have never experienced anything in those three days. I was suffering with the delirium tremors that I'd never had before.

Every time I looked at the floor of my mum and dad's carpet, there was thousands of spiders running everywhere. Of course there wasn't. It's all in my head. Every time I shut my eyes, I could hear these two Afro Caribbean men having a full-blown conversation next to me and I would open my eyes and nobody be there. It was horrendous. I couldn't sleep because every time I shut my eyes, I would bolt up upright in bed, full of fear. Didn't eat, didn't drink, do anything until the third day. And on the third day my mom said I had some water and I had some dry toast. How you feel? I said, I'm feeling a bit better than I was. Still very, very bad. And she said, right, your dad needs to come up here now because he's poorly, he needs, you need to go in your room. And we said, fine. And I remember she said, you know what you need to do, don't you? I said, I do, I. I need to go back to the recovery rooms, and I remember ringing this guy who had seen around the rooms, he was twenty-five years sober.

Now. Length of sobriety means nothing. It's quality of sobriety that people go for. You can see if somebody's living, living the life or living the lie. And this guy had seen him in loads of meetings and he was on fire. So, I rang him and I said, please, can you help me? And he said, no problem, I'll meet you tomorrow at the Funky Monkey Coffee shop on Davenport where I lived. I'll meet you there tomorrow at half ten.

I'm not. And can you not, can you not pick me up? You bet. No, I can't. You can walk. And it's all about putting the action in and putting the effort in. You see, for years, Alan, I thought that somebody was just going to come and save me. Somebody's just going to come and save me and everything's going to be all right. News flash for James, don't is going to come and save you. Yeah. You have to do this yourself with help. So, I spoke to this guy and I met him at the coffee shop and I met him every single day for two weeks at that coffee shop. I walked up still shaking and shivering like a shitting dog for two weeks and he'd buy me a coffee because they had no money. And we talk and we'd read the book and we'd go through the twelve steps and I remember, I went after two weeks. I remember waking up, I remember thinking.

I don't want to drink and use that obsession had been removed out my head. That thought had gone, so.

Alan:

So, in some ways then, your new addiction was staying straight. You. You had prioritized being a normal human being and giving your mum and dad the love back and getting your brothers etc, and that was your priority. So, you had a new addiction, which was a good one.

James:

Yes. Yeah. So that's exactly what the book says. That's that, honestly. Thank you. Because that's exactly what the book says.

It says we have to replace drinking and using with something else in a positive way. And that's what we do. And that's exactly what you've said.

Alan, you hit the nail on the head. So, I did a. Replace my bad behaviours with the good behaviours of getting clean and sober and living life not just for me, but as you put it there, for my family as well. And I knew I'd done a lot of damage, a lot of damage. And

I had to build all. All these relationships back up. And it takes time, but I was very impatient. I wanted it all now.

So, I remember thinking, after two weeks, I don't want to drink. And that obsession has never returned in over fifteen years and never returned once.

Now let me tell you, it's a graft, getting through recovery is absolute graft. I can't lie. People reading this book now, I can't sugarcoat it and say you're get to recovery and everything's going to be okay, but until it's not. Yeah, it's not all going to be okay. I lost. I've lost some. I've had some of the hardest times of my life in recovery. I haven't picked up because I don't need to pick up. Because by getting into recovery and working through this new way of life that we're granted with, that we're given, doesn't mean everything's going to be okay. We still get comatose, but it just means we can deal with it a lot better. Yeah. That's all it does. It gives us the mental capacity to deal with anything big or small without picking up a drinking drug. That's all it does.

So, I threw myself in recovery, absolutely threw myself in recovery. And I made. I did a very simple thing again, just like I did in two thousand seven. I put recovery number one and my family number two. I had no job, so it was only those two. And for the first eight months, all I can remember in my early eight months of recovery was I slept loads because my body's repairing, because I'd ravaged, rubbished it that much. I was. I was gone. So, I slept loads so my body could repair and all I did.

I would wake up in the morning, the first thing I would do was open my AA book and read and I would speak to people in recovery. As you said, I'd switch from drinking drugs to the new addiction of recovery, getting clean and sober and doing anything it takes, going to any lens to get clean and sober. Because I didn't want to live that life anymore. I was broken. I've got into that much pain. You see, with pain comes growth and you can't grow without pain.

So, I got to that much pain that I could. I can't do this anymore. And that was the turning point for me. The turning point was I thought, I can't do this anymore. So, I threw myself into recovery. And for those first eight months, I slept loads. My mom bought me a PS3 so when I wasn't doing AA stuff, I was just keeping occupied. I've never been a gamer, but she thought it's the best thing. And I didn't work. I was on Bennett. I was on full benefits then, first time ever. And you know what? Life was very, very, very simple. But, you know, even to this, it's the happiest I've ever been. Yeah, happiest I've ever been. Simplest. Didn't have anything but the happiest. And I just really. I just really did my recovery.

After eight months, my uncle, the one that was trying to help me with the electrician jobs, he texted me one day and he said, how would you fancy a job selling cars? And I went, oh, yeah. So, I went. And it was a friend of his that owned two car garages. One was your old bangers and one was your luxury cars. And I got a job, suited and booted, working in the luxury cars. And I'm talking luxury like Rolls Royce's, Lamborghini's, Range Rovers. There were all the top cars. So, I went working with this company, this guy, and I was there just over a year and of course the. The cars, the money, the clothes, that sort of overtook my recovery a little bit. I was still doing my recovery and I was still bleeding sober. But then it became about what I've got.

I ended up getting with somebody new. I left my daughters The mother of my daughter. and this person was also in the recovery rooms. I ended up being with her three for twelve years. And in that time, there was loads of highs and lows, but for the first five years of the recovery, I'd start on a high over the years, and then gradually. Gradually I'd come down and I wasn't as happy as I had been in recovery. And it all goes down to the fact that I wasn't doing Alan, what I was meant to be doing. It's very, very simple. If you do what's suggested, you will have the best life.

If you don't do what's suggested and you can, you think you could do it James's way, your life's going to go pretty in recovery.

So, I got to. And again, a little bit like the. The drinking and using, I kept moving the goalpost. Well, I'm all right. I'm okay. I'm not drinking. I'm not drinking. But I wasn't living life. I wasn't excited for life. And I remember the. The. The. The girl that I got with, she was also in recovery, but she was doing it a slightly different way than I was. And I would see her come home from her friend's house absolutely on fire for recovery. Like, glowing like I was at the beginning, she was buzzing. Buzzing to make new friends. Buzzing for recovery. Buzzing for God. She was just on fire. She was lit up with life, and that made me. Seeing her made me go, I want some of that.

I can only describe myself at that time as I was lukewarm. I was in my recovery. I was doing just enough to scrape by daily. Wasn't happy, felt something was missing. This was five years clean and sober. We'd moved in together; we were going on holidays.

We had my daughter every Wednesday and every weekend. She had a son who became my stepson. Raised him since he was about eight years old, nine years old, but just something was missing. And then.

I remember going to Chester where she used to go visit her friends and speak about recovery with the girls and remember I got invited to go when I spoke with the boys and. Yeah, and we were chatting and stuff, what they were saying, I didn't really get. It was from the same book.

Anyway, it ended up that I said to this lad, can you take me through the work again? Because that's not uncommon for. To go through the work a few times, the twelve steps, you. You revisit it and it's like a little bit like a refresher course.

So, I said to this lad, can you take me through it again? They said, no problem. And when we went through the work, when we started the work on the first session, the first session was three hours. And when we started to work, me, him and another lad.

I Came out of his house with the same feeling. I'd seen my partner on fire. I was like, where's this? This feeling was incredible. And I was five years sober. And then what I've done is I've been. I've built on that. That feeling for the. For the last ten years, for recovery and for God has never really left me. I've been on fire. The same fire as what I saw my partner at the time with.

Alan

Did you just say for God?

James

I mentioned a little bit earlier. Okay, so with the twelve steps of recovery, it speaks about God, but not as God as in the Christian God or the Muslim God. It's not in the AA book to make it inclusive.

For your belief, they say, use a God of your own understanding, if it Makes sense to you. That's all that matters. Yeah. Now I've been brought up, I was way, so my granddad was a Catholic, my mom's a Catholic, and, but we, we're not practicing, we're never practicing. We, we, we just believe now. I've always believed since being a little boy in God. Never had a relationship with God.

Until I came out of my friend's house and I got, I got back, back on fire for recovery and for God. That's when I sort of my, my, my walk with God took off ten years ago. And, and that, and it was a perfect, perfect question because I think that's one of the reasons why I was lukewarm, because I wasn't building a relationship with a God that would help and guide me through my recovery journey.

So, I got on fire for recovery, even from God.

I really. And I did what I did at the beginning, five years previous. I put everything in it. I put everything in it. I thought, you see, one of the main things of recovery is working with others. So, once I've gone through the twelve steps and I'm clean and sober and I'm living my best life, which I was, I then have to pass that on to the next person that comes through the rooms that's still suffering. That's the deal. Yeah, that's the deal of the twelve steps. You can't get, you can't get well and then off and see you later.

You have to give back? It's part of the process and it's ironic, you know, because the more you give back, the better you feel.

So, the more I was giving back, the healthier in body and mind I became and more, was revealed and then I decided, and then what happened was me and my partner at the time we broke up and I threw myself into church, found this church, threw myself into church. Within a few months of me going to this church, it was Christian church. A few months ago, going to church, I got baptized and I gave my life to Jesus. And that was on the twelfth of twelfth of April, twenty fifteen. So, it was just after I'd been lit up for God. Sorry, just after I've been lit up for when I went through the work again. And from that point I have then, over the last ten years, I've then built this relationship with a recovery with God. So, at this time I was working for, I'd been. And got a main dealer work. I was working for Volkswagen. So, I was working for a main dealer selling cars. Had left the other job and gone into this.

I think we wanted to move and. And it wasn't the. Obviously, the money wasn't guaranteed. It was a little bit cash in hand and whatnot. So, we wanted it proper. So, I was working up at Volkswagen, and I was doing really, really well and we just kept going to meetings, build, building on the recovery.

Life was good. Life was good. I can't really think of anything that sort of, sort of happened in that time. I remember. Yes, I can.

So, I remember not long after I got baptized. Twenty fifteen, my daughter emigrated to Canada with her side of the family, her mom and their side of the family and to live out there. So, we're going out there. She left school, she was fifteen, this was in twenty fifteen, and she lived out in Canada. And we'd speak every day on facetime. Obviously, it's six in the morning, it was eleven o' clock at night there, so we'd facetime. I was on the way to the gym, but after three months of being there, I had an absolute breakdown. I had a meltdown at work. Never drank and used, but I had an absolute meltdown because I was just missing it.

I ended up going on the sick for a few days, ended up having a few words with a boss which weren't pleasant, and ended up leaving and going working for another Volkswagen dealership. And after about a year of my daughter being in Canada, I remember just before her sixteenth birthday, she. We'd facetime all the time and she rang me on this particular occasion and she said, I want to come home. And I said, charlotte, you. You're there with your mum and your family and stuff and you, you're in Canada, you're living your best life. No, I'm not, Dad. I walk home, I miss my friends, I miss you. I miss my side of the family. I want to come home. So, I said, well, I need to speak to your mom. Spoke to him when my mom said, she's sixteen in a few weeks, if that's what she wants to do, fine. So, my dad paid for me to get a flight over to Canada, spent a week in Canada. It was.

It was incredible. I was. I said to my daughter, why do you want to come back to Manchester again? It was absolutely lovely. Anyway, brought her back and we ended up that I wasn't with this girl. We were always splitting up, getting back together, splayed up, getting back together. And it ended up that in twenty sixteen, when I went and got my daughter My dad, me. My parents had another house that was empty. We used to remember Grandma's house and she died. So, me and my daughter moved in and my dad said, that's your house now. Right, fine. And it was just me and my daughter for twenty sixteen. And it was incredible. It was ace working at Volkswagen. She was at college. We're having just me and her. And I remember thinking, Alan, I remember it was only five years ago where I weren't even allowed to see her.

I wasn't allowed to see my daughter because it was an absolute nuisance. Now we've got our own house and I'm the sole guardian, the sole custody of my daughter. Her mum stayed in Canada. Yeah. How does that happen? These are the joys of recovery, of building relationships back up where you're a trusted member of society

So, I ended up getting my daughter back and she's living with us and it was amazing. Off she was to college and work.

Life was good. Then we ended up getting back with this girl. She ended up moving in and. And it was. It was good for a good number of years. It was good. We got married in twenty eighteen and in Twenty nineteen. My dad passed away through the same illness as what I've got, so he died in mine, in my mum's arms.

I Didn't pick up, didn't have a day off work or anything. Didn't go on the sick. Just cracked on with life. Because that's what I was saying before, because life still treats you, you still get thrown at your butt. I had all the tools to deal with it through recovery. Not wanting to pick up, not needing to pick up.

I was building my recovery network Corp. I was building great relationships back up, my family and my partner, because we just got back together and just got married and everything was going great and then lockdown happened. So now we're at April twenty-twenty, Because I'm vulnerable because of my COPD I was the first to leave work and I remember in lockdown.

I start. I had no social media at this time. This is the birth of JT motive. I had no social media at that time. But what I did have was where I had WhatsApp and at the time you could do thirty second WhatsApp statuses. So, I started to put little motivational videos on for thirty seconds and it only goes to your contacts in your phone. Yeah. I kept getting messages off people going, these are brilliant. I look forward to these. And then it ended up there. Because in domestic fat, in lockdown, the first couple of months of lockdown, domestic violence went up twenty-five because people were at home, they were drinking more, they were under, they were spending more time together than they usually did, and everything went a bit haywire. I always say there's two types of people in lockdown. Those that got fit and those that got fat. Now, I was one of the ones that got fit, doing the Joe Wicks on the TV and stuff like that.

We did the garden open, if you remember. The weather was gorgeous, it was boiling. So, we, I us as a family. I love lockdown. Five months. I was five months off work, getting paid more money than I was if I was in, which was strange. But anyway, life was good. But my phone was off the hook. People ringing for help, asking for help. So, I ended up opening up a YouTube channel, calling it JT Motive and putting videos on there to help people in recovery. Then they did it with Instagram, then I did it with Tick Tock, then I did it with Facebook. So, this is how the birth of GT Multi was built in lockdown to help people overcome addiction because there was social distancing, we weren't allowed to contact and. And that's how JT Motive was born. And then I built sort of my recovery platform on social media to help people. And I was doing this and working full time at Volkswagen after we went back from lockdown and I just remember building JT Multi book, getting the tens of thousands of followers, helping people. People would message me saying, can you help me? I can't stop drinking or I can't stop using or. And we would chat and I would point them in the right direction, and we'd build this community, really this family, this community of people that we all stuck together, and we all helped each other on social media and people would leave and join. It was great. This still goes today.

I remember I was working it. So, after lockdown, I worked at Volkswagen Bolton. I'd moved from Wigan to Bolton. and I was very good at what I did and I sold a lot of cars and I got treated well from management because I was very good at what I did. So, I didn't start till ten where everybody else started at half eight. I had my own office, and I had like a manager's office, which was just for me. Not a lot of them were sales. I'd like that because I got this preferential treatment. But where they're selling four cars a week, I'm Selling four cars a day. So, my boss is like, Tim, you can do what you want. Yeah, you can come, come whenever you want, go whenever you want because you could because you're doing the numbers. And I remember in twenty twenty-two I became number one again. See it again, not drinking but getting these awards because of obviously excelling. And I got number one in the country again in twenty twenty-two. And then in twenty twenty-three was the start of the breakup of my partner that my ex-wife.

Now we broke up in twenty-three because we used to pop loads on social media and social media can be very Fictional, should we say? People only put the good stuff on; they don't put the bad stuff on. And when we split a lot of people would say, I'd never guessed that from what I see on social media you must be very, very careful what goes on social media. So, we ended up splitting but there was for the last two years from twenty-twenty one to twenty-three, it wasn't great, it wasn't great at all. There were loads of crap showing on both sides.

There's stuff now I, I can think of stuff now when I say this to me to hide it. My partner. I regret doing that. Like I worked, I worked constantly. My phone was on, I would sell cars on my days off and my ex-partner used to say, you're off your days off or you're on holiday, switch your phone off. And I go no; I'm not doing that. I would never give all my time and that's one thing I regret and I've learned from that. And I do that today when I want time with my, my grandson or hi, I switch my phone off or I leave it upstairs and go down so I can spend quality time because if it's there I'll pick it up because I know what I'm like.

We ended up splitting in twenty twenty-three and it ended up being that the JT motive I sort of stopped doing. I put it on the back burner. I do the odd one now and then, but my head was in bits with it all.

I had to leave the church that we both went to together because we both went to the same church and I had to leave that church because she can't continue to go. I didn't want to cause any upset and we do the same meetings as well. So, we had to find different meetings. We had to sort of like rebuild a new little structure for myself and then it ended up that in twenty twenty-three again I ended up getting with, with Heidi, and do you know what I found, Alan? I found. I kept apologizing all the time. I was apologizing to her all the time by thanking her all the time. And she was like, what are you thanking me for? And I was like, just because of what you're doing. She said, yeah, but this is normal. I never knew that. Yeah, I never knew because I was so used to this toxic relationship I was in for the last two years. Well, he was toxic for two years at the end. So, I ended up that we. We got together. Everything's going amazing. Still is to this day, which is obviously two years in, still going amazing.

At Volkswagen, I became number one in twenty-two dealerships and then Volkswagen start to take a bit of a turn. Started to. I started to not hit my numbers and head wasn't in it.

Last year, when my brother rang me, I've got. I've got a stepbrother, a middle brother who's my. My older brother's best friend and he's been part of the family since he was sixteen. And he rang me and he said, I've got your job. And I said, I've got a job. And he said, no talking on building sites, sharing your story and helping people just like you do in JT motif. So, this is how I became a motivational speaker.

He put me in touch with his company, and I did my first talk in April twenty fourth, I did my first talk for ISG, but now I got into administration and they did my first tour there and it's just snowballed from there. Going on sites, talking to people, talking to boots on the ground. Because suicide on construction sites is the worst ever. Two a day.

Seven hundred nineteen SUICIDES in the construction industry from 2022 to 2023.

Alan:

Yeah. And there's only about three hundred deaths from accidents, so it's double the amount suicides as opposed to accidents.

James:

It's horrendous. And even though people like me, and I've got others, my friend, circle of friends on LinkedIn who go out and do the speaking, like yourself, we're just scratching the surface.

There are so many blockades. I speak to big CEOs through LinkedIn, and their words are to me, Alan, we don't need your services. James, we don't have a drinking drug problem.

Alan:

That shows you that they are not aware of the current and ongoing situation and that they not in any understanding, by any way, shape or form of who we're working for them and the pressure that they are under.

They're not in the real world.

James:

They're not in the real world because it's absolute rife. Doesn't matter where you go or what you do, it's rife and, and that's experienced. When we go to ours. When I went to my first talk, at the end of the first session, one guy come over to me, the end can have a word, and he told me his life story that he'd never told anyone. And I'm. And, and he, I helped him and his misses cut down the drinking.

So, me doing these, speaks of these talks. I go, and it's now transpired where without. We're now going in Europe now. We've been invited to go to Europe, fly out for the week and speak to construction sites for the whole week and then fly back. Alan, it's incredible. Yeah, it's incredible that. You see, I've always said I've got thirty years' experience, I've got fifteen years in addiction, active addiction. I'm fifteen years in, in recovery and if I've got all this experience and I can't go out and share that with someone and use that experience to help the next person, then I'm being selfish.

I mean, exactly like yourself. Yep. We go out and use it to help people.

Alan:

I've just got so much to give. I've been in construction forty-one years, and I've seen it all, literally seen it all, even down to not long ago, hearing a very senior manager say to other senior managers, if you don't like it, you know where the fucking door is. Right. Whilst only hours before, the office manager was putting all posters up about mental health first aiders and Christmas is coming. This is the time of year when men need to talk, open up. So, the same company, by default, who are trying to tick boxes, are not believing what they say. So, and that's what the idea of this is about.

James:

So, do you think we'll ever break that? People like me and you?

Alan:

I think we need to carry on the good fight. I think, I think that there's still the obstacle of, if you had a bad kidney, a bad liver, you would ring your boss and say, look, I'm not feeling so well. My liver's playing up on my kidneys. But you won't if your brain's playing up. But ultimately your brain is still an organ that you've got no control over. And like taking vitamins for your kidneys or your liver, you can start to try and control your brain. But you. You need help and you really do need help, and it needs to be encouraged. So that's how I feel about the whole situation. But if we don't try, then we never will.

I have recently spent time working in the Netherlands and while posters were being put up in the tea break area about mental health and supporting each other, some senior people were using words like, if you don't like it, you can fuck off.

So, there is still the massive element of box ticking to win work, we need to keep pushing for there to be a change in mind set and belief.

James:

No, correct. We have to keep trying.

Alan:

If someone in 1939 didn't start Alcoholics Anonymous, you, my friend, would be dead. And no doubt someone who started that spoke to his friend one day and went, do you reckon we'll ever make a difference? So, let's live by the theory between me, you and any other motivational speakers that we are going to make a difference. And that's what. That's. That's what's going to make us. Make us carry on fighting the good fight.

I just want to put out, if you can, quickly, anybody reading this now at the end? Anybody? You've come to the end. Thank you so much for reading my story.

James:

It's very difficult for me to put my whole life in an hour and a half. There are loads more. There are loads more I've got. But just to let people know out there, there is support groups out there.

Like Alcoholics Anonymous, Cocaine Anonymous. You've got one called Andy Man's Club, which I haven't been to, but I've put people onto and they are now clean and sober and living the best life.

There's lots of different support networks out there, but I say it all the time, nobody's going to come and save you. You have to put the work in yourself. And if you go to one of them and after a few months nothing happens, you think it doesn't work that go and try another one.

Don't just then give up.

You have to keep going and putting yourself forward. Because if you keep going, I'll end on this, if you put minimal into your life, you're going to get minimal out. Yeah. If you put loads into your life, you will get loads out. It's just the way it works. Yep.

Alan:

I will list a few of the support networks in the back of the book James.

I say as well, the same amount of negative energy is the same amount you use as positive energy. So let the negative side go instead of looking out the window and going, oh, it's a beautiful day. Oh, but it'll probably rain this afternoon. Just think, it's a beautiful day. I'm going to take my jacket with me and if it rains, I'll get on with it. That's it. Simple as that. And it's just a thought process change. So, we've got our all work on it. We've all got our battles every single day and we carry on doing what we do for everyone. So, all good?

Thank you, James, I can’t thank you enough for helping with this project.

We both have the same passion for supporting others.

www.jtmotiv.com

https://www.instagram.com/jt_motiv?igsh=OGczY2F1bWExMHV1&utm_source=qr

https://www.linkedin.com/in/james-ford-jt-motiv-96b38530b?utm_source=share&utm_campaign=share_via&utm_content=profile&utm_medium=ios_app

Chapter 30: Beigal Bakery in Brick Lane

Archway Dal

We moved to the Archway in Islington North London in 1970.

I'd lived in about 6 other places including Canada before I was 8 years old and finally had somewhere to call home. Within a few days I'd made friends with some local kids who I'd end up with for the next 20 years or so.

We were all into football and although we lived in Islington most of us went arsenal one week and Tottenham the other as we were too young to go to away games. Over the next few years, we would get up to more than the mischief other local kids were and we were always seen as the local troublemakers. By 11/12 we'd wait around the top of Holloway Rd waiting for the coaches leaving Highbury and scream and shout at the Northerners making their way home.

Then one day someone decided to throw a half brick at the coach So now we had found a new game for Saturday evening.

Over the next couple of years, we'd all decided which of the two teams we'd rather follow.

I chose Tottenham with a couple of others while most decided on Arsenal.1975 I'm 13 and decided to go to my first away game out of London, Coventry City away was my choice.

I'd admired the older blokes who always seemed to be at every home game and defended the club against any away fans, I thought they were as special as the players big brave lads who didn't care how many away fans were coming out onto Tottenham

High Road, they were always willing to get stuck in. So that's who I started to try and be noticed by.

Getting noticed by these blokes wasn't easy like I thought. It wasn't until the following year when I was noticed at a home game I can't recall who it was against but as usual I was hanging around the Corner Pin pub after the game with the guys I looked up to and suddenly there was away fans all around us I had a choice, Fight or Flight I decided to fight, well I was small and never the world's greatest fighter so I took a good few punches but when it was finally over the older guys were happy to talk and suddenly I'd made a whole load of new mates.

By now my home life had reached a really bad place both my parents were shit,

Mother was an alcoholic and Dad was a gambler and womaniser who thought nothing of literally punching both me and my little sister absolutely anywhere the punch would land. It was at this time both me and my sister were put into Dr Barbados children's home for 9 months and to today I know that's where my mental health issues began.

This was 1976/77 things were different back then and children's homes were a hive of perverted care staff preying upon children without any chance of getting caught.

Sadly, I fell victim to this just to protect my sister as I was told if it's not you it's going to be her.

So, I think that's had a profound impact upon my life and given me serious trust issues.

After 9 months of sheer horror in the home we went back to living at home with our parents although not great it was better than where we had been.

Life at home was actually ok as I was just left to my own devices come and go as I pleased.

Football became my life my friends at spurs were my family now and every week I'd be outside the pub meeting up with my little group of mates or alternative weeks you'd find me sitting at the top of the escalator at Euston Station or some other London train station waiting to travel so some god-awful city up north. It's now 1977/78 Spurs are in the 2nd Division Honestly, it's my favourite season I've ever had. I managed to go to every game home and away in the league the first and only time I've done that Memorable highlights.

Charlton away we took 1000s most probably close to 10,000 and rumours were flying around Millwall were coming in big numbers. I was in the giant side of the ground and watched as Millwall tried to steam our fans but came completely unstuck as our numbers were just huge and they backed away.

Mansfield away the first time I'd got a real hiding at a game It couldn't have been a worse day weather wise it'd rained from the moment we arrived at the Station in the grim East Midlands town.

Absolutely soaked we made our way to the ground about 10 of us.at about 14.00 we saw a local pub with what looked like a little firm outside and thought yeh that's them and running at the pub punches started flying now I've said I've never been a hard man or the best fighter in the world but I just loved getting involved but this day I realised at 15 years old taking on Coal Miners was probably not a great idea. Suddenly I came face to face with what looked like Desperate Dan from the comics I'd used to read **BANG** I smashed him with a right hook flush on his chin and expecting him to drop instead he shook his head looking at me and said Is that it!!!!!! Crack I felt my jaw as his shovel-like hands kept pounding me until I think he lost interest and moved away.

Lesson learned definitely that day.

Southampton away our last game of the season and a draw was enough to get us promoted back to the 1st division not much happened but one of the best days ever at football that season. It was about this time my parents moved away from Archway to a little sleepy town in Essex Halstead.

I had no choice and moved with them but absolutely hated it and them even more for forcing me to leave the area I loved. I made friends with some great guys but spent most weekends back in London going to football gigs and staying with my lifelong friend JD whose mum made me so welcome.

I eventually had to leave Halstead as I started getting nicked for stupid stuff and building a bad reputation for myself.

I moved to Woodbury Down Estate and lived with my Nan I think my mental health started to really start affecting me not long after moving there.

My Nan was fantastic I could do no wrong despite getting nicked a couple of times for minor stuff at football she never criticised me and I realised how bad my parents actually were the beatings I'd suffered from my father since about 6/7 years old where a thing of the past and I for the first time in my life I had unconditional love.

In August 1979, I made it into the national press Stoke City away, always lively as Stoke had a really good firm We'd arrived early in Stoke about 8 of us and a bloke I didn't really know but I'd seen at a few games. Outside Stoke Train Station we were spotted by a little firm who came steaming into us.

It wasn't a great big row I'd been in loads worse just a few punches exchanged and it just broke up. About 14.30 4 hours later we walked through the turnstiles into the away end looking forward to a good game. Straight away I noticed a couple of the Stoke firm we'd had the row with earlier in the day standing with half a dozen Policemen pointing in our direction Suddenly I'm grabbed handcuffed and dragged away. It turns out the Stoke fans had grassed us up to the police moaning they'd been beaten up and wanted to press charges.

Unbelievable they'd come unstuck and then gone running to the police. So off we go me and a bloke called Tony to Stoke police station to be charged and what I thought would be bailed to appear at a later date in court. To my surprise we were refused bail and sent on remand to Risley Remand Centre in Warrington, this remand jail was so notorious that everyone knew it as Grizzley Riley.

It was a bank holiday weekend so we were held until Tuesday morning when we were taken back to the magistrate court in Stoke. I was found guilty of assault and fined £522.50 bear in mind this is 1979 it was an absolutely huge amount of money most probably 10 times the normal fine for fighting at football and the following day our pictures were in 2 or 3 of the national newspapers telling the British public what scum we were and how we ruin football for everyone.

As usual Nan was sympathetic and blamed the police for locking up her poor little grandson for 3 days.

Over the next few years, I got arrested to many times and the last time was lucky not to go to prison. On a Friday I'd been in Tottenham Magistrates Court and given a suspended sentence of 1 year for cheque fraud.

The following day we played Forest at home and I was trying to stay away from any trouble, at half time we were having a quiet pint under the park lane stand. Just minding my own business, the police came storming in as there were fans from both teams climbing up on the partition that separated us. It was nothing to do with me and after the previous day I really wanted to stay out of it, but everyone was pushing and shoving towards the police and with my pint in hand I'm pushed from behind and the contents of my pint go all over copper, next thing I feel a crack on the back of my head from a truncheon and I'm grabbed and nicked once again. I get bailed and I'm told to attend Tottenham Magistrates Court again on Monday morning. I spend all weekend thinking about my suspended sentence I'd got on Friday and I know I'm going away for at least a year on Monday.

So off we go I said goodbye to my Nan and head to court. I'm found guilty and stand there waiting to be sentenced while my previous is read out by the clerk of the court. He gets to a conviction about 5 months earlier and stops the magistrates have a chat and I'm fined £75.00 for criminal damage to the officer's uniform

Nothing mentioned of the suspended sentence I'd received on Friday Thank God for pen and paper before computers my conviction from Friday hadn't been updated on my record a massive sigh of relief and in reality, the start of the end of running around the country being a little Herbert.

It's now the mid-80s and I really start feeling like my life is going up and down more often than normal compared to many friends, my mood swings are getting worse at times and I start to think of suicidal thoughts for the first time in my life.

I feel I'm always being looked at and people are judging me about everything I do.

I totally remove myself from friends and family and get married to what was a lovely girl but it doesn't work out as I'm completely paranoid, not about her but about myself and being judged and within 2 years it's over.

We'd moved to Spain together before we split up and I decided it's a good idea to move back to England. On a night out I bumped into an old friend in the Beigal Bakery in Brick Lane who invited me to a party the following week.

It was there I met some new people who've become my friends ever since. It's now the early 90s and a couple of them are doing the Knowledge to become London Taxi Drivers and in 1992 I decided I'd do the knowledge myself. This is the most stressful thing I'd ever undertaken and at times I become very depressed about if I'd be able to complete it.

I went to the doctors and was put on a short course of antidepressants for the first time in my life and sadly not the last. In 1995 I became a London Taxi Driver the proudest day of my life up to that point. My life started to look better I had a really respectful job people admired cab drivers back then.

A year later I met and fell in love with Alison who is the mother of my 2 beautiful daughters. We ironically moved away from Canonbury to Halstead the place I'd hated years before as we wanted to buy a house and somewhere nice for our children to grow up. It was now as a father I really encountered mental illness so badly it's affected me badly to this day.

Being a parent I had unconditional love for my daughters and began to think how did my parents treat me how they did and pit us into that nightmare Children's Home where I was sexually assaulted time and again. I became so angry, but I held everything inside although it was eating away at me, I still hadn't ever dare to mention what was making me feel like this to anyone: I must have been weak I must have deserved it. I must have asked for it All thoughts that went through my head little did I realise that none of it was my fault and it was years until I faced up to that fact that I realised I was just one of thousands of young children who were assaulted in children's homes by evil predators that preyed on us.

After spending a couple of years in Halstead we moved back closer to London to Chadwell Heath where we stayed for 5 uneventful years. we moved back out again this time to a beautiful town Hockley still staying in Essex which had now become my home county. It was here although very happy I really with hindsight started on the downward spiral that would eventually lead me to trying to take my own life in May 2014. It's funny looking back but I don't think you personally see or feel the signs of your own demise as it creeps up on you without warning. It's little things I look back on now that I can see I was suffering with some form of mental illness, I'll give you an example One night at work a passenger left a really nice pint glass in my cab. Lovely I thought, little did I know that having nice pint glasses was to become an obsession I'd aim to finish work in London and head out towards home approximately 50 miles away and I'd plan my route to visit as many pubs with beer gardens in the front and collect as many glasses as possible. This resulted in roughly 400 glasses in my garage over 18 months, absolutely ridiculous for what I don't know, I had more glasses than most pubs and I'd spend hours scouring Essex pubs.

In around 2010 I'd say that I started to withdraw from my family life constantly at work or at home in bed. I'd completely lost all interest in life altogether but thankfully I was still providing for my family and paying our mortgage. My eldest daughter about this time was taken ill and spent the best part of 18 months in and out of Great Ormond Street hospital which put tremendous stress on both me and my partner as one of us had to be with her while the other one was at home with our youngest daughter. 18 months of sheer hell watching your flesh and blood in horrendous pain and multiple operations actually breaks you mentally if you're already struggling.

Once she was better and thankfully, she's absolutely fine now I threw myself back into work but suffered a shoulder injury which is where my real problems started. I had to have minor surgery on a rotator cuff injury which is fairly common, but I became addicted to the pain relief medication Tramadol which was prescribed to relieve the pain. 8 tablets a day is the maximum dose but within weeks I was taking 15 to 20 tablets a day and drinking 10 cans of Red Bull each and every day. I hid it all from my family and friends and like a fully functioning alcoholic nobody was any the wiser. This carried on for roughly 2 years until things really started to unravel.

In early 2014 I went to Africa with my younger daughter who accompanied me to a tiny village in the motif Ghana where we helped set up a computer program for school children and clothing program to help children be able to attend school. My partner hadn't wanted our daughter to go as this place was very rural and not very sanitary to say the least but I insisted that it'd be ok. Well, it wasn't she was taken very ill after 10 days with E. coli poisoning which meant an emergency dash back to the UK and a trip to hospital. Rightly so my partner was furious with me for putting our daughter in danger and refused to talk to me for weeks. Then in May I was in bed pretending to be asleep which I was doing on a daily basis now just because I felt safe tucked up and not having to deal with the real world.

Early in the evening there was a commotion downstairs, getting out of bed I went down into my daughter's bedroom to find water everywhere, now I don't know why to this day but I started screaming shouting at everyone especially my eldest daughter whose room it was that it's her fault etc etc. She was in absolute tears but I continued to rant and rave at her my partner and eventually I smashed my fist through the bedroom door, which abruptly seemed to bring me to my senses. The girls spent the night with their mum downstairs in one of the bedrooms I'd just gone up ebbed and left them to it, what a terrible father I'd become.

The following morning nobody spoke to me but at the time I really didn't care. By Wednesday the atmosphere in the house was awful everyone had gone out to either work or school and I was alone with just my thoughts. I decided to mow the lawn stuck in my headphones and spent the next few hours with my mind racing away how much better off they'd be without me. I went in and out of the garage it must have been 20 times and rigged up a rope with a noose in and out time after time not knowing what to do. I sent a goodbye message to Alison and finally found the courage to leave this world behind. But I just couldn't do it and within minutes Alison was back home and I was a crying heap on the floor of the garage She proceeded to call an ambulance because I was obviously having a mental breakdown. While she was doing this, I found the courage to do what I'd intended all along I got on the ladder placed the noose around my neck and kicked the ladder away Alison who was on the phone to the ambulance service had come out to the garage at that exact moment unbecomes to me and started screaming There were two builders working next door or opposite I'm not totally sure but they came running and immediately cut me down.

The ambulance and the police arrived soon after and I was taken to Southend Hospital. I spent the next 12 hours in A&E before being transferred to the Mental Health Unit at Basildon Hospital.

After spending a couple of years in Halstead we moved back closer to London to Chadwell Heath where we stayed for 5 uneventful years. we moved back out again this time to a beautiful town Hockley still staying in Essex which had now become my home county It was here although very happy I really with hindsight started on the downward spiral that would eventually lead me to trying to take my own life in May 2014. It's funny looking back but I don't think you personally see or feel the signs of your own demise as it creeps up on you without warning. It's little things I look back on now that I can see I was suffering with some form of mental illness, I'll give you an example One night at work a passenger left a really nice pint glass in my cab.

Lovely I thought, little did I know that having nice pint glasses was to become an obsession I'd aim to finish work in London and head out towards home approximately 50 miles away and I'd plan my route to visit as many pubs with beer gardens in the front and collect as many glasses as possible This resulted in roughly 400 glasses in my garage over 18 months, absolutely ridiculous for what I don't know, I had more glasses than most pubs and I'd spend hours scouring Essex pubs.

In around 2010 I'd say that I started to withdraw from my family life constantly at work or at home in bed. I'd completely lost all interest in life altogether but thankfully I was still providing for my family and paying our mortgage. My eldest daughter about this time was taken ill and spent the best part of 18 months in and out of Great Ormond Street hospital which put tremendous stress on both me and my partner as one of us had to be with her while the other one was at home with our youngest daughter. 18 months of sheer hell watching your flesh and blood in horrendous pain and multiple operations actually breaks you mentally if you're already struggling. Once she was better and thankfully, she's absolutely fine now I threw myself back into work but suffered a shoulder injury which is where my real problems started. I had to have minor surgery on a rotator cuff injury which is fairly common, but I became addicted to the pain relief medication Tramadol which was prescribed to relieve the pain. 8 tablets a day is the maximum dose but within weeks I was taking 15 to 20 tablets a day and drinking 10 cans of Red Bull each and every day. I hid it all from my family and friends and like a fully functioning alcoholic nobody was any the wiser.

This carried on for roughly 2 years until things really started to unravel. In early 2014 I went to Africa with my younger daughter who accompanied me to a tiny village in the motif Gahna where we helped set up a computer program for school children and clothing program to help children be able to attend school. My partner hadn't wanted our daughter to go as this place was very rural and not very sanitary to say the least but I insisted that it'd be ok. Well, it wasn't she was taken very ill after 10 days with E. coli poisoning which meant an emergency dash back to the UK and a trip to hospital. Rightly so my partner was furious with me for putting our daughter in danger and refused to talk to me for weeks.

Then in May I was in bed pretending to be asleep which I was doing on a daily basis now just because I felt safe tucked up and not having to deal with the real world. Early in the evening there was a commotion downstairs, getting out of bed I went down into my daughter's bedroom to find water everywhere, now I don't know why to this day but I started screaming shouting at everyone especially my eldest daughter who's room it was that it's her fault etc etc She was in absolute tears but I continued to rant and rave at her my partner and eventually I smashed my fist through the bedroom door, which abruptly seemed to bring me to my senses. The girls spent the night with their mum downstairs in one of the bedrooms I'd just gone up ebbed and left them to it, what a terrible father I'd become. The following morning nobody spoke to me but at the time I really didn't care. By Wednesday the atmosphere in the house was awful everyone had gone out to either work or school and I was alone with just my thoughts. I decided to mow the lawn stuck in my headphones and spent the next few hours with my mind racing away how much better off they'd be without me.

I went in and out of the garage it must have been 20 times and rigged up a rope with a noose in and out time after time not knowing what to do. I sent a goodbye message to Alison and finally found the courage to leave this world behind. But I just couldn't do it and within minutes Alison was back home and I was a crying heap on the floor of the garage She proceeded to call an ambulance because I was obviously having a mental breakdown. While she was doing this, I found the courage to do what I'd intended all along I got on the ladder placed the noose around my neck and kicked the ladder away

Alison who was on the phone to the ambulance service had come out to the garage at that exact moment unbecomes to me and started screaming There were two builders working next door or opposite I'm not totally sure but they came running and immediately cut me down. The ambulance and the police arrived soon after and I was taken to Southend Hospital. I spent the next 12 hours in A&E before being transferred to the Mental Health Unit at Basildon Hospital.

So, I'm in Southend hospital after attempting to take my own life, lots of tears and anger directed especially at the builders that had cut me down. I assessed by various doctors firstly for the damage I've done to my neck and throat and then by a shrink. It's determined I'm a danger to myself so I'm going to be transported to Basildon Mental Health Unit. I honestly remember nothing of the journey but clearly remember entering the building, it reminded me of entering Risley Remand centre many years earlier.

We went through a big set of doors with security staff in attendance but the next set of doors were shut and wouldn't be opened until the doors behind us were shut firmly. I was then escorted to one of the wards where I was to be held until deemed safe to return home. I was taken straight to a room which was to be my home for the next 2 weeks. About 07.00 I'm wide awake and decided to have a little wander around but I find the bedrooms are in a closed part of the ward you can leave your room to get to the bathroom but your locked in a secure area throughout the night.

I met a decent guy while in there I only spoke with him because he was dressed decently in what I'd describe as casual clothing. His name was Tom who was living in Greys but actually came from Shepherds Bush originally and was a QPR fan. We were both in there for the same reason. The first week was dreadful queuing up for meditation that'd been prescribed was literally like something out of the Movie One Flew Over the Cuckoo Nest. You'd get in like give your name to the nurse and wait while you medication was put into a little white pot. You were then passed it through a little hatch with a nurse standing right next to you Once you've taken it you've got to open your mouth wide and the nurse checks you have swallowed all the tablets. For 5/7 days I was feeling like a zombie with all the medication I was given. You don't actually feel like you're being questioned by the staff it's very relaxed and just feels like a very easy chat between two people but with hindsight they are assessing you constantly. There were some very strange and some very sad people locked up with me

A very young girl 15 who should never be on an adult ward was escorted by two nurses 24/7 and even monitored throughout the night with her bedroom door held open and a nurse sitting on a chair just watching her while she slept very sad as she'd tried cutting her wrists and self-harming herself since she was 10 years old a very messed up kid. We also had a brass in there who was a heroin addict who was having heroin delivered by friends who'd smuggle it in for her. Like everyone in there she suffered from anxiety and depression and was a regular visitor to the unit as many were.

After about 10 days it was decided that I was eligible to be released to the safety of my home as they knew my partner and children were at home. So, my release was scheduled for a few days later. I was then told my partner had told one of the doctors that once I was released, she'd be leaving the family home immediately so my departure was in jeopardy. On the morning of my scheduled release I was really worried about her statement because if there was nobody at home my release would be in jeopardy. But for once I was very lucky the doctor, she'd spoken to hadn't spoken to the nurse who was responsible for my release. So, after 14 days locked up, I was released and literally ran out of the hospital grounds and jumped into a passing taxi back to an empty house in Hockley.

My partner had gone taking my two daughters to her sister's house in Tamworth. I didn't see them for a week until they eventually returned home. My two daughters were both very different in their attitude towards me my eldest who I'd verbally abused the night of my breakdown was still not talking to me at all and my youngest daughter was weary but was still very loving. I had home visits every two days from a Care in the Community nurse for about two weeks and then I was left to my own devices other than the regime of medication I'd been put on. After a few weeks I was back to work and totally out of the blue I received a text one morning from my partner telling me after 18 years she was leaving me that day and had already found a place to live. Don't bother rushing home as we are leaving in the next 5 minutes. It absolutely breaks my heart I've not spoken to my elder daughter since that morning 11 years ago, I've tried but my number was blocked.

So, for the second time in my adult life, I'm single but this time I'm a father and my heart are broken because of my children. My relationship with my youngest daughter was still broken but not destroyed and over the next few months we managed to slowly rebuild it and I have the greatest relationship with her to this day. We had to sell our beautiful home with me walking away with about 15% of our clear funds so my partner had enough to put a roof over the children's head. So, I started my life from zero once again.

My mental health was at rock bottom although taking my tablets every day I still felt suicidal and spent hours thinking of ways to get it over with as the best way out of this torture. Tablets Drowning Crashing Into a bridge Hanging Cutting my wrists You name it I spent hours contemplating my own demise. About 18 months later I got a message from an old girlfriend who I hadn't seen in 30 odd years but had always stayed in contact with every few years by post card phone call or most recently social media. She had been living in Spain for many years and was heading back for a few days to England. I said we should meet up for a coffee and have a real catch up.

So, in December 2016 we met at Braintree Train station and headed off for that catch up.

So now I'm meeting up with my first love after over 30 years big problem I've got a date that night with some random bird off plenty of fish dating app. But things go really well and I forget about that and spend the night talking with Michelle and then the next 4 days together before she fly's away to India for her holiday. We spend all day and night on the phone while she's there and we arrange I'll fly to Spain on Christmas Day.

So, begins 7 years together getting engaged then married and finally getting divorced in May 2025. So where does that leave me now. Well life is very hard at times I still have those crazy thoughts running through my head but I've found help with that by originally contacting the Samaritans, they were absolutely amazing I spent many many hours talking with councillors about my life my problems and my coping mechanisms which were non-existent to be honest. But I've learned that I'm not to blame for what happened in Dr Barnados as a child and the blame lies solely with those who abused me and also with my parents who were negligent in their care for allowing us to go there in the first place. I now feel I'm able to talk what happened without fear of people looking down on me for being weak and knowing where to apportion the blame.

It's crazy to think I held all this in for 40 years when if I'd not been ashamed and had been able to seek help earlier many of the nightmares, I've lived through may have been easier to cope with. Now I still have problems I don't think they will ever go away and on the rare occasions I bump into my father I can't help myself but look at him with distain, but I cope and most recently I've actually started helping on the phone line for those who've suffered like myself but haven't yet worked out how to deal with it. I'm no councillor I just listen and help them with phone numbers like the Samaritans who have access to the right people.

Taking the right medication also helps with my anxiety it's a daily struggle but one that I can now manage and look forward to the rest of my life hopefully helping others. Alan thanks for asking me to write this up it's actually really helped although tough at times it's actually very cathartic. I know some of the things I've done in life haven't been good or seen as normal but for a kid with my background I'm pretty sure by the end which hopefully is many years away I'll of left just a small mark on some people that has enriched their lives. I'll now strive to make life better for those on the edge and tell them You have to reach rock bottom before you can climb back up the ladder but you can make it if you try.

Chapter 31: Demons & Goals Colin W Chelsea Diver

Firstly, I would like to thank Alan for asking me to write in his book about what I have been through over the last 7,8 years and giving an insight of what I went through with my health.

I first felt that something was wrong with me about 8 years ago, I was finding it hard to settle at night I couldn't sleep to a regular pattern properly and being a postman that what I didn't want or afford as I had to get up at 3.30am in the morning.

I was getting agitated with things revving up on people for no reason at all and arguing out on the street telling customers to fuck off.

I knew that I had to try and sort myself out but as time went on it was becoming worse I would go home from work and about 8pm 9pm I'd run a bath and start to find I just couldn't face to get it was as though a panic attack was coming on I would get into the bath I'd hardly got in it and something was brewing inside of my head and had to get out panic was taking over my head and it was a terrible feeling I'd get into bed only for a few minutes later it would come on even stronger I had to get out of bed and at this point it was getting worse I thought if I went for a walk that it would calm down.

I found myself walking around Salisbury at 2,3,4 o'clock in the morning only to find that when I got home to put the key in the door I couldn't go inside I would pull the door shut and have to go out walking or sitting on a bench to try and calm my demons down what was going on in my head I honestly put my worst enemies through it you cannot guess to know what it's like during the day you're doing your job of work and thinking was it going to happen again that night I was trying to work out what was causing it to happen at that time I was going through a lot of personal shit and finding myself getting messed up on Facebook about the illegal immigrants that were coming to our shores grooming our children and raping them and robbing our elderly that really took a hold of me which didn't help it was taking my life over I knew I have to try and keep off it ,in one incident at night I was out walking late at night and I thought I would ring 111 and see if they could advise me on any help that was out their they asked me a lot of what was to me silly questions about my symptoms I was telling him about it all and all of a sudden the chap said are you by a river because he could hear running water I said yes I am sat by a river his reply right don't do anything stupid and jump in I told him I'm not that at that point he said please move away from the river and that was going to get me an appointment with a psychiatrist and he would ring me back in 5 minutes so he rang of and rang me back within in 5 minutes saying that he had booked me an appointments in a months' time my reply to that was are you taking the piss a fucking month I said you was meant to be helping me not prolong things and put the phone down on him.

I told my partner and she said why don't we go on holiday to see if that would help me so things were booked to go to Cyprus looking back on it now it turned out to be for me a nightmare I'm not one for sunbathing so all day I was following the shade of the parasol and at night my demons were back twice as bad with the heat of day and night I couldn't rest it was like you couldn't get enough fresh air through your nose always felt like three quarters of it was blocked up I was waking up at 2 3 4 o'clock in the morning still not being able to settle I took to walking around the hotel and just trying to get my head down for a few minutes in any corner or crack I could it was like a torture for me I was beginning to think where the fuck is all this going to end the whole holiday I never slept at night and was walking around my partner who I can't praise enough was so supportive I couldn't of wished to of had anybody better at my side she was a true partner and I can't thank her enough but the demons would still visit at nights when

I got back off of holiday I booked an appointment with the doctors I went along to see and have a chat with him and told him what I was experiencing he said you are over loading your brain and to relax and take time to distress your brain by reading a book do puzzles and staying of Facebook and just to chill out anytime I got 10 mins I tried doing this but still my demons wouldn't leave me even socialising I couldn't rest I would be in a pub talking to somebody and it felt like a demon was on my shoulder telling me to lash out to who I was talking at the time put a bottle over their head or even put a glass into them terrible thoughts thank god that never ever happened.

All of these experiences are still fresh in my mind as if it was yesterday I remember a friend of mine called Steve Greenwood, I was telling him what was happening and told him that I couldn't get to grips with it I told him about my chat with the doctor and what he said about reading a book, puzzles and listening to music I said to him over a laugh that I'd soon be on who wants to be a millionaire with that advice, Steve said when he went through something similar he went for a run and tried to break the breathing patterns thought he was taking the piss as he is a bit of a prankster I imagined looking like David Bedford the old long distance runner with tee shirt and headband on running around a football pitch at 3am in the morning but as it was I had to try it one night as I was really having a terrible time with it that night so about 11pm I set of from my partners house across the road to the football pitch at that time I was reaching 60yrs old now people coming home on the last bus looking out the window must of thought what the fuck is that bloke doing this time of night running around a football pitch it did the trick for about an hour I was breathing heavy like a pea do in a playground so again I had to go for a walk until I was exhausted.

When you're living with the partner, she must think he's at it with another girl keep going out late at night, one New Year's Eve

I had to go out again which was now playing on my mind what she must be thinking.

At this time I also noticed that I was struggling to complete my postal delivery at work I mentioned it to people to see if they was feeling the same but like me, they just took the piss but it all came to an abrupt collision on the 20th June 2020 which was a Saturday evening I'd been and had a few beers with my mates in the club in the afternoon usual crack but when I got home and had something to eat I found that I could chew but couldn't swallow my food I had to keep going to the bin and spit it out, I told Paula that I needed to get some fresh air into my lungs and go for a walk down to the local park & ride shelter I was sweating like mad I thought it was due to the heavy coat I had on this time it was about 11.30pm I was sat on the bench planning a route I could take and try and walk things off I only managed about a 100 yards when something was telling me to go home and get up the hospital.

I got to a certain point and my demons was telling me to run home but sense told me to take things steady when I reached home Paula said you look terrible and she would take me up to the hospital we packed a bag and set off when we arrived and booked in the receptionist told us we could have a 3,4 hour wait we told her we expected that so after being booked in I was called to a room and asked to explain what was going on with me she informed me I would need an ECG on my heart with that I was taken for the ECG and kept in a cubicle for an hour a doctor came back and told me the results it wasn't good news unknown to me I had suffered a stroke and I wouldn't be going home and I was being kept in hospital for further test the next day he said that it was the best thing I had ever done in my life to come to the hospital.

After talking to a specialist in hospital he told me until they were happy with more test to be done I would be staying in hospital, until they were happy to let me go home well that period lasted for 6 weeks that was due to covid and they didn't want to move anybody from hospital to hospital so my day was once I had taken my medication in the morning that was my day over and just had to just lay on the bed that was ok for the first couple of weeks but it got very boring was very fortunate that my partner Paula was allowed to come in each day to visit again she was a real Trojan standing by me.

I had gone from Sailsbury, to Poole to Southampton to Bournemouth hospitals, I thought about the demons and how I would cope if they came back to haunt me sometimes I found myself walking around hospitals at stupid o'clock but where I was sleeping during the days it wasn't to bad boredom again was the main thing to cope with I eventually got moved to Southampton where I had to have a quadruple by- pass to my heart people say you'll be fine when the op happens which was the case but the night before you wonder and worry if it went wrong the surgeon came to see me the night before and talked me through the procedure the reason it had to be done was my heart was solidly blocked I was told my 6 specialist that they was amazed I was still alive and that was how bad it was.

Going back to when I was in Southampton hospital one night I couldn't rest again so I went for a cuppa and found myself in the lift around 3am in the morning with some old guy going for a coffee as Costas was open 24 hours the old boy asked me what I was in for and was it heart problems he could make out the dressing and what I was hooked up to he said if you fancy a chat and a tea come and find me I thought oh fuck I can't be doing with that but I took pity on the old boy and went and found him sat down with him and started chatting I told him about my demons and what I'd been through the early morning walks not being to open the door when I got back home he said Colin the thing wrong with everyone in life nowadays is they don't take time to have fun they don't de-stress themselves they just work, work, work for what ? to pay bills meet deadlines pay mortgages he said before his wife died they would take themselves of two stately homes and wonder through the gardens he said his wife lived for flowers and that was their way of chilling out and making a calmer life for themselves he still did it as a promise he kept to his wife after are cut we said our goodbyes and never saw each other again but I have never forgotten his wise words about finding something good in your life that you can focus on to try and de-stress your head which I was trying to do I was telling this to Martin King who was phoning me every day Martin was a massive Chelsea man in every way.

He was a tough man, scared of no one and when he was with you, you knew that you could fight off an army, but deep down he had a heart of gold and we was good friends my first chat ever with Martin was a bit of an eye opener we had just come back to Tottenham court rd. to a pub their it there was quite a few us as we'd just come back early from West ham he grabbed me by the arm and gave me a dressing down saying he'd seen me about a few times and said I was welcome in their company but if ever I let them down you'll never be able to associate with them or drink around Chelsea no problem I said thanks for giving me the shake down he got to be a true friend every day he would ring to see how I was and if my demons and gone away it was a very sad day and great loss to know that he'd passed away a few months later I was talking to another Bernie Marsh and he said Martin liked my company and that I was to be thought as one of the gang now which I thought was an honour to be told that

The surgery on my bypass had gone well but it felt like I'd been 12 rounds with a double decker bus ,bruised very sore and aching I felt shattered I asked the nurse before I had the op if I could take a good luck charm with it was a key ring with my partner's little granddaughter the nurse sad before you go into surgery I will tape it to your wrist which I couldn't thank her enough ,again I couldn't thank Paula enough she was an absolute rock driving down to Southampton and different hospitals to see me and bringing little Miyah with her really gave me a massive boost on the way to my recovery she never knew what was going on in my head before the op with my demons as I didn't want to scare her, as the days went on the nurses showed no mercy in getting me up and about saying if I wanted to go home I'd have to get of my arse and put some effort in to get home if you've had a bypass op they get you in a chair get a tea towel for you to fold up and use kind of a teddy bear and holding it close to your chest and trying to get standing without holding on to the chair and just clutching your so called teddy, fuck me that really hurt but morphine was at hand if you needed it I eventually I got strong enough to go home that was a bollocks up because they forgot to order my taxi back to Salisbury so being pissed of you play up as our kind do they eventually got me a cab and that was it I was going home to Paula and little Miyah, there is nothing that beats being in your home surroundings with your loved ones close to you.

When I got home I thought that all my troubles were over but one day whilst sat watching the tv in the afternoon I put my hand to my left eye to wipe my eye and found that my vision was very bad and that seemed to only 30% vision I shouted to Paula who was in the garden o explained to hear what had happened and she said I think we should get up to the hospital to get it checked out to remember it being a Friday afternoon late she duly rang the hospital and they told us to get up to the hospital straight away they kindly kept the eye clinic open for us until we had been seen I had a quite intense test done on the eye and said that they was going to send me to Poole hospital the next morning to see a specialist so the Saturday morning we set of for Poole again I was given a good two hours of test and scans and dyes put into my eye the specialist told me that I was correct to go to hospital but she wasn't a specialist in the findings she had come across and was referring me back to a specialist at hospital in Salisbury Monday morning I thought things was moving very fast so my thoughts was theirs something very wrong on the journey home again I wiped my eye and could only see 10% vision witch was a little bit scary so what was left of the weekend I spent worrying as to what maybe wrong, Monday morning came and I saw a DR BLACK he wasn't happy with the eye and said he was going to get me booked to see several specialist later in the week I came home with Paula and explained to her that my vision consisted mainly of pink and green psychedelic flashes going in my eye the day came to go to the hospital to see the specialist one told me that at the back of the eye I was experiencing minute strokes to my eye

Another specialist said I had blood cells that needed to be zapped by a laser beam to break them down so now I was getting very concerned I went and sat down with

DR BLACK for a chat he said when he had gathered all the information he would contact me in a couple of days I caught the bus back from hospital into town I went round to Tesco's to get some shopping while I was their my phone rang and it was DR BLACK saying that the results were not good and that I must go down to Bournemouth hospital immediately he had just come of the phone to a specialist friend of his and said myself and Paula must come down together as a life changing decision had to be made as soon as possible we couldn't go then as we had to pick little Miyah up from school the specialist told us that we must get to Bournemouth the next day straight away fuck me I thought now what's going on Paula was worried as so was I everything goes through your mind now what could be more worse than just having a quadruple bypass about a month ago, again the next day we set out for Bournemouth hospital with an appointment with a specialist at the end of our journey we arrived at Bournemouth and checked in the receptionist gave us directions and said the specialist was waiting for us ,we was shown to her office she talked us through what was going to happen again a lot of tests and dyes put in the eye we were shown back to her office she had a colleague with her do they read out the results and said it's not good news colin the bare facts of it all is if you don't come back first thing in the morning will be dead this time tomorrow fuck me talk about a bomb being dropped, she said it is as simple as that that's why we had to call you both in to discuss what we've found and the decisions you and Paula had to make to me it was a no brainer other than to have the operation she said you have a blood clot heading straight to your brain and it will take your life to seemed as if you was in a tumble dryer your heads being thrown about everywhere we both got in the car back home to Salisbury even though Paula was talking to me I couldn't help but thinking of the shit that was going on in my head I've got to get a will make sure she was taken care of and I could feel the tears trying to come the thought of not seeing and little Miyah again choked me up inside but I had to fight back my emotions that night was full of what needed to be done the next morning ,the next morning again we set of for Bournemouth for surgery the operation that had to be performed was called a carotid endarterectomy they had to open my neck up and insert a cow's organ into it to allow blood to keep flowing to the brain and hopefully keep the clot where it was lodging it so I was prepared for the op and wheeled down for surgery again I asked if a photo could be put under my pillow of little Miyah as she was my little angel watching over me

When they took me down to the holding bay before you get wheeled into theatre the anaesthetist said I'm pulling this op your blood is draining from your body and your pulse is going down I said to him please don't I've signed the DNR I know what the outcome will be if you don't let me go through he said I'm going to talk to the surgeon who came through and spoke to me and said it's up to you if you want to go ahead with it by now the drugs they put into me and numbing my neck were taking hold on me my last words I said to him please I'm begging you don't stop it and then I was out for the count and wheeled into theatre that was the only time in my life I've ever begged for something, when I woke up from surgery I couldn't swallow I was panicking like fuck I do also remember in a dream or whatever it was a was falling backwards in a sea of water and trying to reach out for help all in grey surroundings all off a sudden I saw this fantastic bright white light above me and trying to take me upwards at that point I could hear people shouting at me and slapping my arms face and legs tr6to wake colin colin wake up I could hear nurses panicking I eventually saw 6 nurses around me panic over thank god they said I told them about the images I'd seen and of the bright light they said that was the sign of you going to heaven I still couldn't speak hardly again I was panicking I wanted to sit up but they wouldn't allow it I had to lay still I wanted to punch any fucker that wouldn't let me sit up I couldn't swallow because of the drugs still they asked me if I wanted an ice lolly to suck on I had never been so pleased to have an ice lolly as I did that day it was like Angel's pissing on your tongue ,after 2 hours they allowed me to sit up that was heaven the drugs weren't wearing off but the head was getting itself together a bit I got wheeled onto a ward and kept ask for

Ice lollies to get the swelling down a bit I thought I never ever want to go through that again I'd rather have the bypass than that.

After my carotid endarterectomy operation in Bournemouth I had to stay in Bournemouth hospital for a week to recover the food there was absolutely disgusting there was nothing that you could eat would aid you on the road to recovery the surgeon said you must eat to build your strength up but no way if you ate it all you would get no strength from it one day I asked the porter for a bowl of porridge when they brought it in to me and I just looked at it and I thought fuck eating that shit so when they had gone out the room I opened the window and fucked it off to the pigeons on the lawn below even they didn’t seem keen on eating it on my walkabout around the hospital I noticed there was a Carvery the other side of a fence in the car park I thought if I could get through the fence I'd be ok and be able to get something decent to eat so one day I set off for the car park fence there was some ground work going on in the car park so I thought workmen don’t usually give a fuck to what the damage so I eventually found a hole in the fence which I could squeeze through and got into the carvery and get some decent grub which I needed when I used to get back to the ward the nurses asked me where I had gone as I'd missed dinner I told them a tale that I'd been for some fresh air which they used to except my week seemed to drag and drag the last day I was there and due to be released I asked the nurse I asked the nurse if she could check my dressing on my neck I asked her to check it as it didn't feel right ,the nurse said I was right to get her to check it as indeed it have gone wrong and was infected

So again I had to stay in Bournemouth for a second operation on my neck but this time I knew what was going to happen but that didn't stop my demons from visiting me I must admit they weren't visiting me so much maybe be it was because I had so much going on but if there is anything I can say to anybody for advice it would be stay positive fix your thoughts on positive things like I did and do now, mine is to look forward seeing little Miyah and Paula I'd like to thank all my friends at Chelsea for helping me through it all,

Martin King RIP, Bernie Marsh

Chris Tuddenham, Steve Gaffney, Tristan Tipper,

Gary Holding, Steve Doyle,

Paul Routledge, and my best friend Kevin Rattigan and all from the Willow.

I have been given the all clear to travel by myself now after all this time and can start looking forward to seeing them again, please stay positive and as I did only try and think of positive things.

I only try to things of seeing good friends who care, family who love me, days out and precious time spent.

Everyone out there is dealing with something, no matter how big or small.

If you need help, please ask, look for assistance and stay strong.

Chapter 32: ADAM, MIND BODY&SOLE.

Where do I start?

I've been meaning to write this for a week, and Alan, I apologise for the delay. But here goes, me

friend. Buckle up and enjoy.

I remember how it all began—going to City home games with my old man from a young age. I

recall some young kids asking for a few quid to watch the car while it was parked. The smell of

chips wafting from the stadium is a memory I cherish—those moments with my dad, just us.

Then, around 17 or 18, I thought it was cool to go to the games with him, but I was wrong. If I had

stuck to our original ritual and not strayed down the wrong path, everything would have been so

different. I got into the wrong crowd—easily led, some might say. But it was Manchester in the

'90s and early 2000s, and I was just 18. We all think we know better at that age.

At 18, I was going to games with a group of lads, some older. We drank until our livers couldn't

handle it, then moved on to drugs—that was inevitable. I'd spend my weekly wages in the blink of

an eye at the stadium—buying a few bags, drinking copious amounts of beer. I lost my iPhones and money more times than I can count. And as I write this, I realise I lost myself too.

My mental health has always been fragile. Growing up, my mum and dad split when I was young.

My earliest memory is of my dad throwing one of my mum's many boyfriends out of the house.

She was an alcoholic, and I remember waking up to her chugging wine straight from the bottle in

the fridge. What hope did I have? This affected me deeply—I just wanted to be loved, but felt like

a pawn in a chess game. My nan, God bless her soul, raised me.

Back to football—I worked 9 to 5 in retail in the city centre for years. I hated Oasis and the Stone

Roses, which might be sacrilege for a Mancunian, but it is what it is. I partied six days a week;

there wasn't much else open worth going to. Yet, I travelled home and away, watching City and

living for it.

Mentally, I was just blotting it out with drink and drugs—living a party lifestyle I now realise I

should have sorted out. But my addiction swallowed me whole. My love life was chaotic—I was

going through women like I was a Casanova. I apologise for the heartbreaks and lies, but that was

my addiction, and it ruined everything. I have a son, born in 2010, who I don't see and isn't even

on the birth certificate because she didn't want him to know what a waste I was.

City was my home, my safe space, my life. Suicide was a constant presence—my burden

alongside addiction. It was either drink to forget or attempt to end it all. I've tried to take my own

life more times than I can count. From tying a belt around my neck to jumping in front of trains—

every method I could think of. But I couldn't do that to the driver or passengers. I overdosed on

my 21st birthday after my ex left me—35 paracetamol and enough drugs to kill a small horse. I

woke up in pain.

My last attempt was in 2017. My ex told me it took strength to kill yourself, and I thought, "I'm not

one of them." So, I set out on a three-day bender—no phone, just money, a lighter, and a dealer's

number I memorised. I woke up in hospital, having failed at hanging myself—couldn't even do

that properly.

That was the start of who I am today. I am the founder of MIND BODY & SOLE, a nonprofit

organisation that has saved me. It's given me purpose—helping others helps me more than

anyone could imagine.

I haven't been to a city game since 2017, though I still follow them, talk about them, and watch

them. It's like the old me—distant. I haven't stepped foot in the city since. I've been sober, only

taking vitamins, thanks to my current partner—my saviour—who looks after me and does everything for me. I don't feel I deserve this life, but I have it. The old me is gone; I've been given a

second chance. I'm not religious or spiritual, but I'm going to try to give this life a real shot and

help as many people as I can.

So, how do I stay on the right path? I meditated a lot during early recovery—probably too much,

honestly. I was like a living Enya album. But it helped, and that's what matters.

I have an addictive personality, and it evolved from drink and drugs to meditation—and then

planting a seed. I moved away from my hometown and settled in a small town 30 miles away.

During COVID, I was walking one day and stumbled across a football club. It brought mixed

feelings—obviously closed like everything else, but I could still smell chips from my childhood.

The love of going to the game was still flickering inside me.

I'll leave it there for now. During COVID, I got into social media—talking daily with fellow City fans

and Adidas enthusiasts. I found a niche in cleaning trainers—buying old ones from eBay and

giving them a new lease of life, just like I was being given.

I found a purpose—helping others during COVID who were struggling with furlough and

uncertainty. We supported each other mentally—just by being there. I shared my story with a few,

and things escalated when someone suggested I start a small business. They offered to help with a logo, and MIND BODY & SOLE was born. It was a risk, but I've never been one to shy away

from that.

Furlough led to redundancy, so I jumped into this wholeheartedly—even though I had no clue

what I was doing. But it took off. Our merchandise became popular, and we helped others with

food vouchers and support.

Back to that football club I mentioned— I finally mustered the courage to contact them and

explain what we do and how I want to help the community. They supported me, got behind the

brand, and I'll never forget that. They don't realise how thankful I am. We now have a stand at the

ground, funded through crowdfunding and a benefactor.

We opened a drop-in centre, where I started going to the ground daily. My addictive personality

was whispering, "Keep going," but in reality, I was falling back in love with the game. I started

going home and away with volunteers—helping out as a kit man and now as head of media. I still

visit the club about seven days a week. We're now an official mental health partner of the club!

It's incredible how much my life has changed. If it can happen for me, I truly believe it can happen

for others.

MIND BODY & SOLE now has merchandise worldwide—from Australia and Canada to Germany and even Whitby. We've helped raise over £20,000 in financial aid since 2022, providing food

vouchers, gas top-ups, and sponsoring a family's mobility car to cover their monthly costs.

MBS saved me. Football killed the old me but also gave birth to the new me.

Lads, we know what it's like to bottle things up. But listen—if I can come out of that dark place

and start fresh, anyone can. We're in this together, and I promise I will always be here for others.

Our merchandise now funds everything we do. We have a fantastic website—

www.mindbodysole.uk—and all profits go directly into helping those in need.

Thank you for reading.

Chapter 33: DARRYL P. USA

To start, I was the type of person who never stopped moving from the time I got up until bedtime. I was up every morning at 5 a.m. I worked 50 hours a week, played softball, and stayed very active.

Then one day at work—what I thought was a typical day—I noticed my legs were hurting much more than usual. I told the guys I was going to take a short break. As I turned to walk to the truck, my legs suddenly stopped working, and I fell to the ground. At first, I thought maybe I had just tripped, but when I tried to get up, I couldn't move my legs. That's when reality hit me, and fear set in.

My boss took me to the ER. The first hospital had no idea what to do, so they sent me to a larger hospital, where I was admitted. At this point, I was growing more worried about what was happening to me. After many tests and spinal taps, I finally received a diagnosis.

The doctor's words didn't sink in at first. That night, sitting alone, I realized I was in bad shape. The "what ifs," the "why me," and the fear of living without the use of my legs kept me awake all night. The next morning, my wife and kids came to see me. Like a typical dad, I smiled and told them not to worry—that everything was going to be alright.

Weeks went by, but still no movement. The doctors decided to send me to an inpatient rehabilitation centre, where more tests were done. I regained enough movement to walk out with a walker, but that didn't last long—I was soon back in a wheelchair. This put a huge burden on my family, especially my wife. She didn't deserve what I was putting her through, and I felt worthless for making her carry so much.

Finally, a specialist diagnosed me with **Transverse Myelitis with MS-mimicking autoimmune disease**, and I was sent to IU Medical Hospital in Indianapolis. I underwent a laminectomy surgery, and the doctor was certain it would fix my legs. For about two weeks, it seemed to work—but then suddenly, my legs stopped working again.

Accepting that I might never walk again was incredibly hard. I slipped into depression and pulled away from my wife and kids. I felt useless as I sat and watched them do the things I used to do with them. My marriage suffered—we barely talked and hardly slept in the same bed.

As time went on, I thought about suicide many times. I became so depressed that I turned to drugs. A few months later, I was served divorce papers. I was devastated and ready to give up. I even planned to end my life that night.

But then my kids came in to talk to me. We sat together, cried, and eventually they fell asleep beside me. Watching them sleep, I realized that no matter what I was going through, I had to pull myself together for them. Even if I couldn't save my marriage, I had to be there for my children.

Time has passed. Yes, I'm divorced, but I've also beaten cancer and regained about 60% of the use of my legs. Since May of this year, I've been living in my own place. I'm not angry at my ex-wife for divorcing me—after everything I put her through, she deserves better than what I could give. In truth, I blame myself and my condition for failing my family.

The one thing that kept me fighting for recovery was my son and daughter. No matter how dark things looked, I always remembered that night we spent together—crying, talking, and hearing them tell me they needed me and loved me. I made a promise to never leave them until the day the big guy upstairs says it's time.

This is how my condition changed my life.

To all the men who are struggling: see your doctor, go to a counsellor, and please talk.

Chapter 34: The Future for Alan Bates

Breaking the Silence – Mental Health in Construction

For many years, I held senior management roles in the construction industry where I mentored young managers and guided team members toward success. Leadership was not just my job—it was my passion. But when illness changed the course of my life, I refused to let it define me. Instead, I invested countless hours in personal growth: completing training courses, studying mental health and resilience, and developing my ability to truly listen. I became a mentor, a counsellor, and sometimes just a voice of understanding for those in need. I shared my journey through presentations titled *"If It Can Happen to Me"*, appeared on podcasts, and contributed guest articles to leading construction industry magazines. These experiences have strengthened my skills in communication, empathy, and motivation—skills I now use to inspire and empower others every single day.

The Hidden Crisis

The construction industry is built on strength, precision, and resilience. But behind the hard hats and steel-toed boots lies a silent epidemic—**mental health struggles that claim more lives than workplace accidents**. Every year, the industry records **twice as many suicides as accidents**. Think about that for a moment: while safety harnesses and helmets protect workers from physical harm, there is little to shield them from the invisible battles raging inside their minds.

Health and Safety: A Success Story

Over the past 40 years, I've watched health and safety regulations transform the industry. Today, companies know that if they don't comply, they won't win contracts. In short, **they have to do it**. And that's a good thing—these measures save lives. But when it comes to mental health, the story is very different.

The Reality Behind the Tick Boxes

Many companies claim to care about mental health. They tick boxes, run awareness campaigns, and add "wellbeing" to their mission statements. But too often, these gestures are superficial. The real priority remains the same: **get the job done, hit the deadline, secure the next project, and make more money**. Meanwhile, workers struggle in silence—battling stress, anxiety, depression, and burnout with nowhere to turn.

Why Construction Workers Are at Risk

- **High-pressure environments:** Tight deadlines and financial penalties create constant stress.

- **Long hours and isolation:** Extended shifts and time away from family take a toll.

- **Cultural stigma:** "Toughness" is valued, vulnerability is seen as weakness.

- **Job insecurity:** Fear of layoffs adds another layer of anxiety.

These factors combine to create a perfect storm for mental health challenges.

My Mission: TALK4STRENGTH

I've made it my life's mission to change this narrative. Through **TALK4STRENGTH**, I want every construction worker to know:

You are not alone. Your life matters more than any deadline or project.

Real Change Starts Here

Mental health support in construction cannot be a tick-box exercise. It must be a cultural shift—a commitment as strong as any safety regulation. Companies need to understand that **a healthy mind is as critical as a safe worksite**. Productivity and profit mean nothing if lives are lost to despair.

A Call to Action

To every worker reading this:

Speak up. Reach out. Your strength is not in silence—it's in sharing.

To every company leader:

Invest in mental health like you invest in safety. Lives depend on it.

And to everyone in this industry:

Join me. Let's break the stigma, save lives, and build a future where mental health is a priority—not an afterthought.

"The strongest foundations aren't made of steel—they're built on care, compassion, and community."

Alan Bates,

Founder of TALK4STRENGTH

TALK4STRENGTH

Empowering Voices and Transforming Lives

The Roads I Walked

If you've made it this far, you've walked with me through the streets of London—the cold pavements where dreams felt distant and survival was the only goal.

You've stood with me on football terraces, where loyalty and chaos collided, and you've seen the choices that led me into a world of gangsters and danger.

You've felt the weight of disease, the endless surgeries, the nights when pain was louder than hope. You've glimpsed the darkness of depression and the chilling edge of suicide—the moment when life felt like a battle I could no longer fight.

That was my yesterday. A story of scars, mistakes, and lessons carved deep into my soul. But it was also a story of resilience—a story that refused to end in defeat.

The Voice That Rose

Today, I stand not as a victim of my past, but as a voice of strength. I am a **motivational speaker**, a **mental health advocate**, and a **guide for those lost in the storm**.

My scars are no longer symbols of pain—they are proof of survival. Every setback became a stepping stone. Every tear became a testament to the power of hope.

I share my story because I believe in the possibility of change, in the courage that lies within each of us, waiting to be awakened.

Through **TALK4STRENGTH**, I have found my purpose: to help others rise, to speak life into broken dreams, and to remind the world that strength is not about never falling—it's about rising every single time you do.

FUTURE – The Movement Ahead

This is not the end. It's the beginning of something greater. TALK4STRENGTH is more than a name—it's a movement. A call to action. A promise that no one has to fight alone.

The future is about **empowerment**, **education**, and **connection**. It's about turning pain into purpose and creating communities where mental health is not a stigma but a shared responsibility.

The 3 Rs Thought Process

Our signature framework, the **3 Rs Thought Process**, is designed to help individuals:

- **Reflect** on their experiences and emotions.
- **Reframe** challenges into opportunities for growth.
- **Respond** with clarity, confidence, and purpose.

This structured method empowers you to take control of your mindset, overcome obstacles, and make informed decisions that align with your goals.

It's about giving people the confidence to speak boldly, to live fully, and to believe that their story matters. Because it does. Every story matters.

If my journey has taught you anything, let it be this: **Your past does not define you. Your present is your power. Your future is your choice.**

Stand tall. Speak boldly. Live fully. And when life knocks you down, remember—you are stronger than you think.

This book may be closing, but your story is still being written. Write it with courage. Write it with hope. Write it with strength.

Together, we rise.

``Your scars are not signs of weakness- they are proof that you fought, survived, and chose to rise again``

Alan Bates FOUNDER of Talk4strength

``The darkest chapters of your life can become the most powerful pages of your story, if you chose to keep writing``

Alan Bates FOUNDER of Talk4strength

``Strength is not about standing tall when life is easy – it's about finding the courage to stand again when life knocks you down``

Alan Bates FOUNDER of TALK4STRENGTH

Affirmations that have helped me.

Hope in the Darkness

"Stars can't shine without darkness." Even in the hardest times, your struggles are shaping the light that will eventually shine through.

Growth Through Struggles

"Just when the caterpillar thought the world was over, it became a butterfly." Pain often precedes transformation. What feels like an ending may be the beginning of something beautiful.

A Reminder of Strength

"You have survived 100% of your worst days." Every challenge you've faced proves your resilience. That strength is still within you.

Gentle Encouragement

"No storm lasts forever." Emotions, like weather, are temporary. The sun always finds its way back through the clouds.

Safety in the Present

"In this moment, I am safe." Anxiety often pulls us into imagined futures—this reminds you to anchor in the now.

Strength Within

"I have survived anxious moments before, and I can survive this one too." A reminder of resilience and past victories over difficult feelings.

Calm is Possible

"My breath is my anchor; with each inhale and exhale, I find calm." Breathing becomes a tool to gently guide the body back to steadiness.

These affirmations are not a substitute for professional care, but they can be repeated daily—like mental mantras—to help soften the intensity of anxious thoughts.

Support Contacts

1. Men Speak Men's Groups CIC

- Website: mensgroups.co.uk

2. Men Health

- Website: manhealth.org.uk

3. Back and Forth Men's Mental Health

- Website: backandforthmmh.co.uk

4. Men's Minds Matter

- Website: mensmindsmatter.org

5. For Men to Talk

- Website: formentotalk.co.uk

6. ANDYSMANCLUB

- Website: andysmanclub.co.uk

7. Men Who Talk

- Website: menwhotalk.co.uk

8. Men's Health Forum

- **Focus:** Mental health awareness, depression support, and wellbeing advice.

These groups are **free or low-cost**, and many offer **weekly online sessions**, so you can join from anywhere in the UK.

ONWARD SHIFT

Vishal Narbheram

Company Name - Onward Shift

Email - journey@onwardshift.com

Website - www.onwardshift.com

LinkedIn - https://www.linkedin.com/in/vishal-narbheram-56bb3a194?utm_source=share_via&utm_content=profile&utm_medium=member_ios

WWW.TALK4STRENGTH.COM

Special Thanks

I cannot thank enough the incredible men who opened their hearts and shared their journeys of resilience. Your courage to speak your truth is a gift to the world—a light for those still walking through darkness.

To those who faced crippling conditions, battled addiction, endured illness, and carried the weight of trauma: **thank you**. Thank you for proving that strength is not the absence of struggle, but the decision to rise again when life knocks you down.

Your stories will inspire countless others to believe that healing is possible, that hope is real, and that no one is ever truly alone.

"When one person shares their story, it becomes the survival guide for someone else."

Alan Bates—

Founder of TALK4STRENGTH

My parting words.

"Out of the silence of eternity, against the odds of 1 in 400 trillion, here I stand.

My existence is not an accident, but a miracle written into the fabric of the universe.

Every breath I take is proof that impossibility can be overcome, that chance itself can be bent into destiny.

So, I will not waste this rare gift—I will live boldly, love deeply, and leave behind a light that reminds others of the miracle they are too.

To be born is to win the greatest lottery of all, and I choose to honour that victory with the fullness of my life."

Alan Bates

www.talk4strength.com

In memory of

Ian Ulvmoen

I know that you are still the best dressed wherever you are.

Rest in eternal peace brother.

The Herd